PUSH

PULL

SWING

PUSH
PULL
SWING

Men'sHealth

THE FAT-TORCHING,
MUSCLE-BUILDING
DUMBBELL,
KETTLEBELL, AND
SANDBAG PROGRAM

MYATT
MURPHY,
CSCS

RODALE

© 2014 by Rodale Inc.

Photographs © 2014 by Rodale Inc.

All rights reserved. No part of this publication may be reproduced or transmitted in any form or by any means, electronic or mechanical, including photocopying, recording, or any other information storage and retrieval system, without the written permission of the publisher.

Rodale books may be purchased for business or promotional use or for special sales. For information, please write to: Special Markets Department, Rodale Inc., 733 Third Avenue, New York, NY 10017

Men's Health is a registered trademark of Rodale Inc.

Printed in the United States of America

Rodale Inc. makes every effort to use acid-free ∞, recycled paper ♻.

Photographs by Mitch Mandel/Rodale Images

Book design by Joanna Williams

Library of Congress Cataloging-in-Publication Data is on file with the publisher.

ISBN 978–1–62336–397–0

Distributed to the trade by Macmillan

2   4   6   8   10   9   7   5   3   1   trade paperback

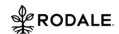

We inspire and enable people to improve their lives and the world around them.
rodalebooks.com

To K and B.

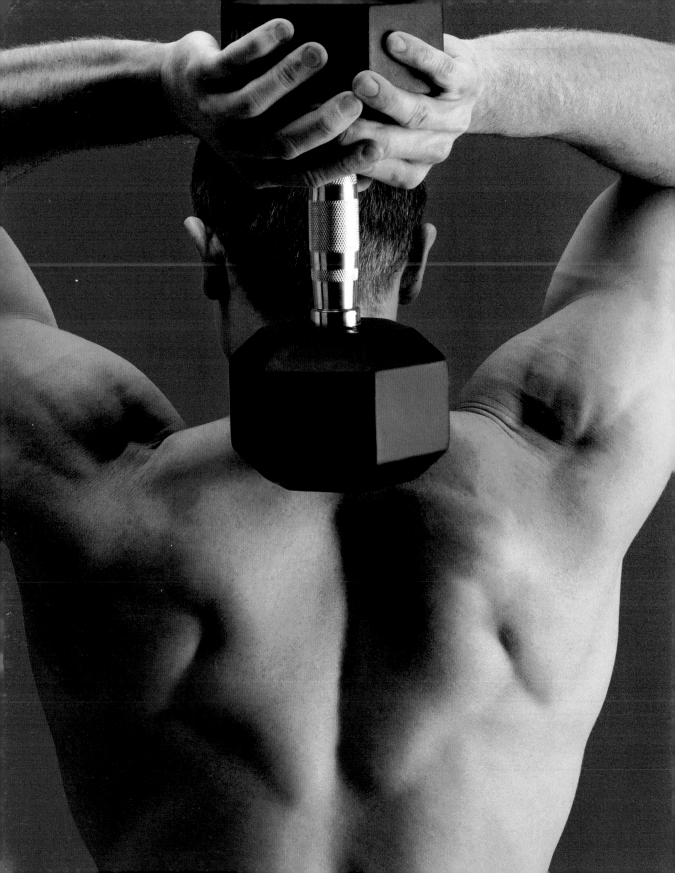

CONTENTS

ACKNOWLEDGMENTS   ix

PART ONE: THE PHILOSOPHY

Chapter 1   3
Push, Pull, Swing
The Philosophy of Movement over Muscle

Chapter 2   9
Dumbbell, Kettlebell, Sandbag
The Holy Trinity of Total-Body Transformation

Chapter 3   19
Old-School Tools
What You Need to Succeed

Chapter 4   27
Your Muscles and How They Move
The Anatomy of Push, Pull, and Swing

Chapter 5   35
Nutrition to Power Your Workouts
Six Steps for Eating Right While Training for a
Leaner, More Muscular Body

PART TWO: THE MOVEMENTS

Chapter 6   45
The Best Dumbbell Exercises
Push, Pull, and Swing with the Muscle-Building King

Chapter 7   89
The Best Kettlebell Exercises
Push, Pull, Swing with This No-Nonsense Work
Capacity Tool

Chapter 8   137
The Best Sandbag Exercises
Push, Pull, Swing for Real-World Strength

PART THREE: THE ROUTINES

Chapter 9   187
The Test Drive
1-Week Tryouts to Learn the Key Moves and
Sample Each Piece of Gear

Chapter 10   193
Build Your Own Push, Pull, Swing Program
Choose a Blend of Movements for Total-Body
Fitness and Optimum Fat Burning

Chapter 11   203
The Workouts
11 Top Trainers' Programs for Dumbbells,
Kettlebells, and Sandbags

INDEX   283

ACKNOWLEDGMENTS

Push, Pull, Swing is the fifth book I've had the pleasure of writing for Rodale Inc.—*Men's Health The Body You Want in the Time You Have, The Men's Health Gym Bible, Men's Health Ultimate Dumbbell Guide,* and *Testosterone Transformation* being the other four. This is the second book that has allowed me to work with Editor Jeff Csatari, my colleague from the early days of *Men's Health* magazine and one of the hardest-working editors I know.

My sincerest thanks go out to every trainer who I consulted during my research, including Tony Ambler-Wright, Lisa Balash, Missy Beaver, Bradley Borne, David Buer, Fabio Comano, Aaron Drogoszewsik, Mike Fantigrassi, Rob Gibson, Joseph Giangrasso, Tony Gonzalez, Steve Hess, Chip Huss, Lorna Kleidman, Annie Malaythong, Ronald Merryman, Erin McGill, Marty Miller, Gabriel Rangel, Prentiss Rhodes, Eric Salvador, Ben Shear, Kyle Stull, Brian Sutton, and David Van Daff. Even though it pained me not to be able to include every one of your workouts due to lack of space, your efforts and interest are greatly appreciated.

A special thanks to the other contributors who made this book possible: Mitch Mandel; Julia Merz; Joanna Williams, art director; Andrew Speer, an owner of Soho Strength Lab who modeled for the exercise photographs in the book; Nikki Weber; Lynn Greenspan; Karen and Courtney Lewis; Troy Schnyder; Stacy Foley; Emily Groff, proofreader (for giving everything her never-miss once-over); Hope Clarke, senior project editor; and the entire Rodale Books publishing team.

Finally, if you learn anything from *Push, Pull, Swing,* you have my dad—a hardcore marine—to thank. He started me on the path to getting in shape so that one day I might do the same for others. Another one down, Dad.

Myatt Murphy

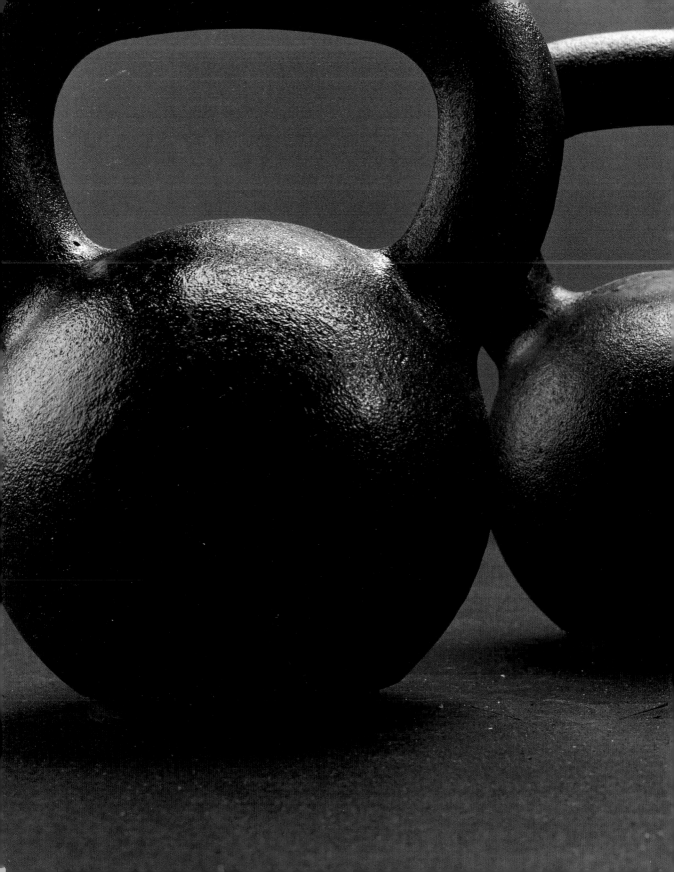

PART ONE
THE
PHILOSOPHY

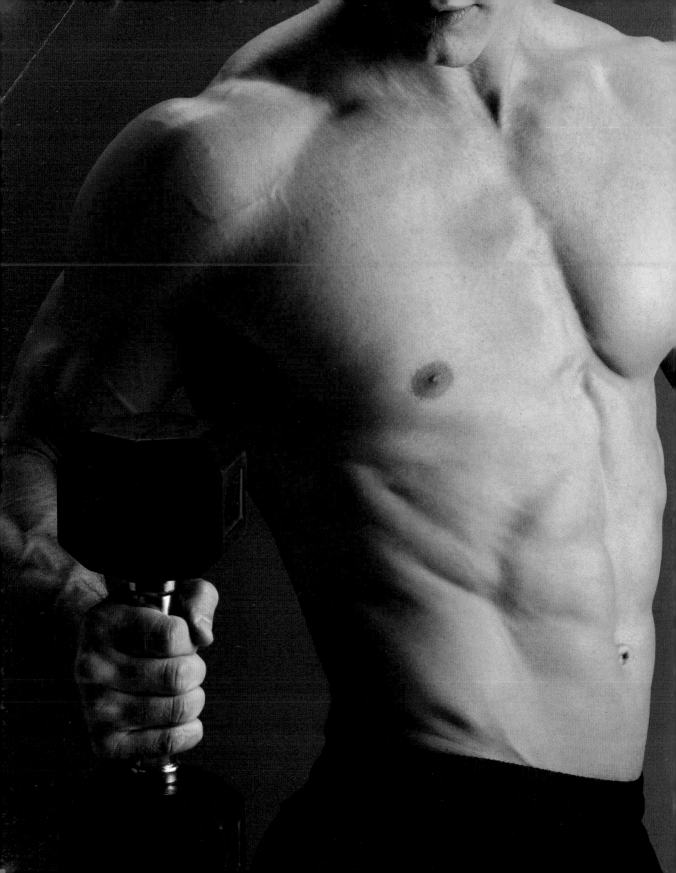

CHAPTER 1

PUSH, PULL, SWING

THE PHILOSOPHY OF MOVEMENT OVER MUSCLE

Please step away from the Smith Machine for a moment and listen to an ancient tale from the Indian subcontinent. Although many different versions of the story exist, the basic gist is this: Several blind men are summoned before the king of a vast land. They are brought into a large room, and inside this room is an elephant. The king asks the blind men to describe the beast, so each man touches a single part of the animal's body. One touches the leg and says, "It is like a pillar." Another grabs hold of an ear and describes it as "a fan." A third strokes its tusk and says it's "like a plowshare."

Each man was sure he was correct. And he was. But when asked to summarize their findings, they could not agree on how to describe the elephant in its entirety. So stubbornly did they hold to their individual assessments that they argued until they came to blows, to the delight of the king.

The story has many meanings. Most interpret it as a parable to discourage dogma, comparing the blind men to preachers and scholars who are blind to new thinking and hold on to old ways.

In one version of the parable, the Buddha ends the bickering with this verse:

O how they cling and wrangle,
some who claim
For preacher and monk
the honored name!
For, quarreling, each to his view
they cling.
Such folk see only one side of a thing.

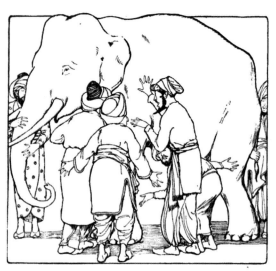
For strength and athleticism, work the entire "elephant."

You're probably wondering what this has to do with strength training. After all, it's rare to find blind men feeling up elephants in a gym. What you do find in gyms, however, is a lot of people who act as stubbornly as those old blind men: They train one way, the same familiar way, perhaps the way they learned 10 years ago from a bodybuilding magazine or a personal trainer. They focus on the vanity muscles, or one style of exercise, or a favorite lift, and as a result they fail to see the bigger picture.

In weight training, there are hundreds of different exercises but really just three basic movements: pushing (which includes squatting), pulling, and swinging. Yet even with so few critical moves, we're always surprised to find that most guys focus primarily on the pushing exercises, ignoring the other two. Take notice of the lifts most guys are doing at any given time in the weight room. Consider your own workout. Overloading your workout with pushing exercises leads to unbalanced training and lopsided bodies, and it cheats you out of

moves that work your whole self more effectively through a full range of motion.

Hey, we're men. We're a little vain. So we curl for bigger biceps, bench for a massive chest, crunch for abs of steel, and squat for powerful legs. But like those blind dudes who each focused on just one part of the elephant, most men ignore the other important body parts during training. As a consequence, their results suffer.

Training single body parts is a really inefficient way to exercise unless you are a bodybuilder preparing for a physique contest. If you want to boost your metabolic rate, burn fat all over your body, and build functional strength, you need to take a grander view during exercise. You need to take in the whole elephant.

Think about strength in practical terms: In real life, your body rarely moves just one muscle group at a time. That would be unnatural. But that's what it does when you perform a Biceps Curl. Ask yourself this: When in real life do you push away from your chest as if you're doing a bench press? Maybe when you find yourself lying on the kitchen floor with a refrigerator on your chest. But that's about it. If you work your muscles in a limited range of motion, you create imbalances in your physique, which in turn can cause posture problems and encourage injury. And you ignore all of those tiny muscles that help move the bigger ones and support your frame.

In real life, your body moves not like the hinge on a door but in three planes of motion, the way a basketball player, mixed martial arts fighter, or regular human being tripping over a curb does, with twists and turns and arms flailing. When you run, swim, jump, skip, tackle, tumble, or dance, you move the whole elephant, not just the trunk. So why train with weights in such a limited way? You're not a fixed joint on a robotic arm in an assembly plant. You're fluid, and so you should train with weights that way. You need to Push, Pull, Swing. If in addition to your favorite pushing exercises you did a mix of good pulling and swinging movements, you would create well-rounded, functional strength for the way you use your body every day. What's more, you'd build a roaring metabolic fire within your body by activating so many more muscles, from tiny to big.

The most versatile tools for doing all three movements are dumbbells, the kettlebell, and the sandbag. Each tool is simple, inexpensive, can be used in a small space at home, and is small enough to hide under a bed. Try that with a Bowflex or Olympic barbells. Most importantly, each one allows you to do exercises using the greatest range of motion.

Take the kettlebell, for example: It's like a cannonball with a handle. Extremely popular in gyms today, this old-school Soviet-era dumbbell allows the user to do an incredible array of pushing, pulling, and swinging moves, plus combination exercises that really challenge your body from all angles. The sandbag offers similar benefits: The sand shifts in the bag as it moves, forcing the lifter to balance the weight, calling more muscle fibers into play for greater functional strength and calorie burn. That's important whether your goal is training for an adventure race like the Tough Mudder, Spartan Race, or *Men's Health* Urbanathlon, or attacking blubber trouble spots like your belly, butt, and thighs.

How Your Body Moves in Three Planes

You already know your weak points, but do you know why they are weak? It's because you're not training your muscles the way they were designed to move. You're inadvertently dissing them by focusing on vanity and ignoring function. To turn that around, it helps to grasp an understanding of how your muscles work in real life—that is, through three planes of motion known as the *sagittal, frontal,* and *transverse* planes.

The best way to understand the geometry of this is to get a little gory. Imagine you're a samurai warrior brandishing a sword capable of cutting a man in two.

▶ You could split an enemy down the middle from the top of his head, between his eyes, and straight down through his spine, dividing him into two symmetrical halves. That's the sagittal plane.

▶ You could cleave him from the side, straight down through his head, shoulders, arms, and legs, until all that remained was a front half and a back half. That's the frontal plane.

▶ Or, you could chop him horizontally at the waist, sawing him into upper and lower body halves. That's the transverse (or horizontal) plane.

Being truly fit, not just strong in a very specific way, takes multidirectional training. By exercising your muscles through multiple planes, the way your body was meant to move, you will find it easier—much easier—to pack on serious muscle, increase your strength, boost your endurance, improve your sports performance, decrease your risk of injury, bring a neglected body part up to speed, and blast off stubborn fat.

Let's look a little closer at each plane of your body.

THE SAGITTAL PLANE, which divides your body into left and right halves, is the most common plane of movement for most weight lifting exercises.

Whenever you perform an exercise that moves your body forward or backward without rotating it or letting your arms or legs cross over the midline of your body, you're performing a sagittal plane exercise. Some examples are neutral-grip Chinups, Squats, Lunges, Stepups, and walking while holding a pair of heavy weights at your sides.

THE FRONTAL PLANE, which divides your body into front and back sections, involves movements that occur laterally and primarily involve your shoulders, hips, and intervertebral joints.

Whenever you move your arm or leg out from your side and away from the midline of your body (abduction), reverse that motion by bringing your arm or leg back in toward the midline of your body (adduction), or move your head, neck, spine, or torso to the side, you're performing a frontal plane movement.

One way to gauge whether you're doing a frontal plane exercise is to flatten yourself against a wall so that your arms, legs, and back are touching it. If you could still do the exercise with all three touching, it most likely fits the bill. For example, wide-grip Lat Pulldowns, Shoulder Presses, Side Laterals (raising and lowering a weight out from your side), Side Lunges, Side Bends, Side Planks, Side Shuffles, Jumping Jacks, and Side-Lying Leg Lifts are all frontal plane exercises.

THE TRANSVERSE (OR HORIZONTAL) PLANE, which divides your body into an upper half and a lower half, is the plane of motion that most people, especially men, tend to neglect. That's a big problem, especially because our bodies tend to work through this plane anytime we twist, turn, bend, or move in all directions. Simply put, any time you perform a movement that includes a rotational motion, such as twisting or turning, you're working on the transverse plane of motion.

The muscles that function in the transverse plane, which include your obliques along the sides of your torso, not only help rotate your body, but they also prevent you from rotating too much, helping your body to decelerate whenever you rotate with any excess force (such as while throwing a punch, hitting a golf ball, swinging a racket, etc.). Just a few common examples of exercises that work along the transverse plane include Chops, Reaching Side Lunges, and Russian Twists.

Focus on Movement, Not Muscles

A lot of guys tend to be body part obsessed—meaning, they have a specific agenda when they weight train, such as increasing their bench press, forging bigger biceps, or finally seeing that six-pack. They use traditional strength training exercises that focus on specific muscle groups and tend to move along the sagittal plane. These exercises typically work what are known as the "mirror muscles," the ones you flex in the bathroom.

But when you spend most of your workout doing moves in any one plane of motion, you can create muscular imbalances, which cause overdeveloped muscle fibers to pull against underused ones. This starts a tug-of-war that often leads to tendonitis, impingement issues, posture problems, and other exercise-related injuries over time.

Even if your body manages to dodge any pain issues, what may not be as obvious is how that imbalance could be holding back your performance—as well as your appearance. Having muscular symmetry has many performance-enhancing benefits, such as keeping your spine aligned. This perk improves your posture, allowing all of your muscles to work more efficiently when transferring power into every movement you make, which could easily equate to having a faster line drive, a stronger backhand, and more power when pushing off a defender, just to name a few examples.

Being an equal opportunity exerciser using the Push, Pull, Swing method can also help you improve upon the physique you already have. Spending equal time developing the muscles behind you also helps accentuate the muscles in front by making your body appear more muscular from all sides. Also, the more evenly matched your muscles are, the more efficient your body becomes at handling heavier weights, pulling off certain intermediate or advanced maneuvers, recovering from workouts of a higher intensity, and burning fat.

Push, Pull, Swing is the solution to the challenge of making your workout routine efficient and egalitarian. In this book, you'll learn exercises that train your body for the way it moves in real life and in sports. You'll find exercises that work you through all three planes: moves that involve swinging and pushing against resistance, swinging and pulling against resistance, or pushing, pulling, *and* swinging against resistance; hip- and knee-dominant exercises; bridges; and rotation-based exercises. Instead of designing your workout around specific muscles, you'll focus on the movements those muscles perform by choosing a balanced mix of pushing, pulling, and swinging exercises and using dumbbells, a kettlebell, or a sandbag for resistance.

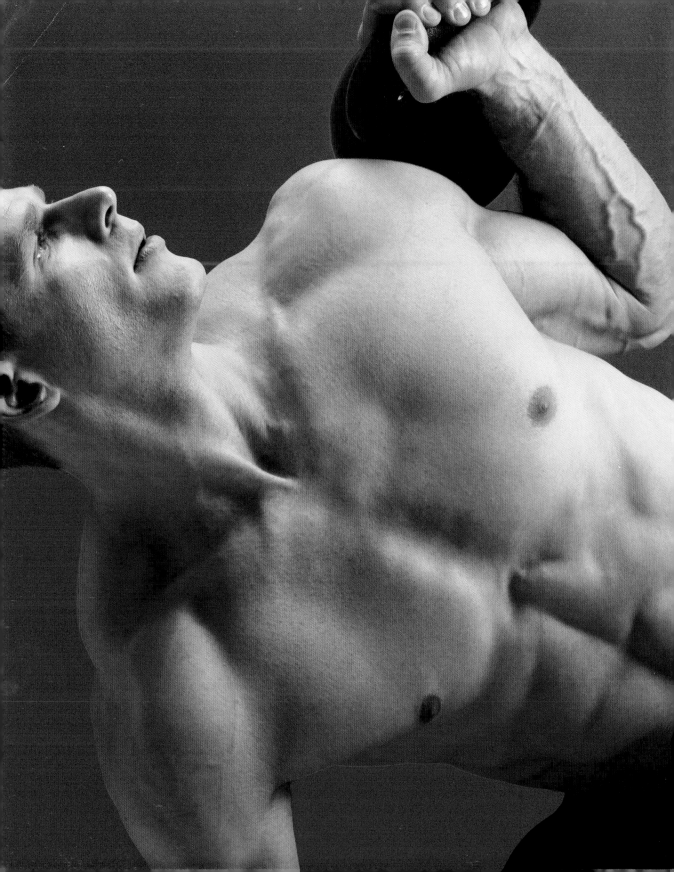

CHAPTER 2

DUMBBELL, KETTLEBELL, SANDBAG

THE HOLY TRINITY OF TOTAL-BODY TRANSFORMATION

Simplicity is the ultimate sophistication.
—LEONARDO DA VINCI

These three simple tools can help you push, pull, and swing your way to a stronger and fitter body. Their small size and simplicity allow for a greater range of motion during exercise, challenging your muscles in ways no other equipment can. You can only go so low, for example, with a Barbell Bench Press. When the bar hits your chest, that's it. But with a dumbbell, kettlebell, or even a sandbag in each hand, you can bring the weight lower, calling more muscle fibers into play and stimulating more growth. That's just one advantage of using a humble dumbbell, kettlebell, or sandbag. Here are more reasons why you should use them for the unique exercises in this book.

They Keep Your Muscles Guessing

Research has proven that muscles adapt quickly to exercise. Perform an exercise for the first time, and you'd better be ready to try something new four to six workouts later, because that's about when your muscles become smart enough to do that same exercise using less effort and energy. When your muscles are no longer being challenged, they aren't growing—and you are wasting your time.

Even the tiniest of tweaks to any exercise can evoke a change that keeps your muscles progressing. And that's the neat thing about this muscle-making trinity. It's hard to tweak an exercise machine (or even a barbell) beyond adding more weight or changing the height or angle of a bench or cable, but dumbbells, kettlebells, and sandbags allow you to make hundreds of technique adjustments, both large and infinitesimal, that work your muscles differently.

They Fit Every Body Type

If you've ever felt uncomfortable performing some pushing, pulling, or swinging motions when using certain exercise machines or performing barbell exercises, the reason could be your unique shape. That's because many exercise machines are built to accommodate an average-size person. But what if you aren't average? If you are short or tall, have long or stubby arms or legs, or have shoulders that are very wide or very narrow, your shape puts you at a mechanical disadvantage on the machine, making certain push, pull, or swing movements awkward or even painful. Dumbbells, kettlebells, and sandbags, on the other hand, work with every body type because they aren't in a fixed position like machines or even barbells. Using them, you can adjust your body more freely, aligning your arms or legs wherever they need to be for the most effective push, pull, or swing exercise.

They Can Work One Arm at a Time

Bilateral training is a fancy name for using both arms or legs at the same time to push, pull, or swing. *Unilateral training* is a fancy name for using one arm or leg or one side of your body for exercise. The problem with performing bilateral exercises all of the time, as you do with a barbell or weight-stack machine, is that your weaker limb quits first. This limits your growth and causes muscle imbalances.

If building symmetrical muscles is your goal, the best approach is often one-sided, unilateral exercises, which work each side of your body independently so you can put more stress on the muscles that need to catch up. What's more, unilateral exercises kick your *proprioceptive muscles* into action. These are the mini neurological helpers that intuitively respond to your movements all day long, making slight adjustments to your posture to keep your body in perfect alignment and in balance. Doing a Single-Arm Press, for example, forces your core to stabilize your spine because of the unbalanced weight you're holding. By training unilaterally, you exercise your stabilizing muscles, chisel your core, and correct muscle imbalances, reducing your risk of injury.

Finally, unilateral training keeps your heart rate elevated for twice as long as bilateral training, since training one arm or leg at a time doubles your effort, forcing your body to burn more calories overall.

Individual Advantages

While dumbbells, kettlebells, and sandbags offer many similar muscle-building and metabolism-boosting benefits, each has its own distinct qualities that make it special and ideal for certain tasks. Let's look at each.

The Dumbbell Edge

The dumbbell has been sculpting amazing physiques since the first Greek athletes hefted *halteres,* crescent-shaped stones with handles, back in the 5th century BC. Halteres were originally used as jumping aids: An athlete would swing the weights forward to propel his body farther during a long jump competition.

By AD 200, the Greek physician Galen had published *De Sanitate Tuenda,* a medical text that described the benefits of using these tools to strengthen the body. For centuries afterwards, other people wrote about the benefits of using resistance implements similar to dumbbells, with the most influential being Girolamo Mercuriale.

Considered to be one of the most famous physicians of the Renaissance, Mercuriale published *De Arte Gymnastica,* an illustrated medical text showing chiseled, muscular men lifting dumbbells and heavy sheets of rock, in 1569. Around the beginning of the 18th century, dumbbell training became more popular among men. Even an 80-year-old Benjamin Franklin once credited his longevity to living temperately, not drinking wine, and performing daily exercises with a dumbbell.

So where did the name come from? Historians believe the word *dumbbell* was first coined centuries ago in England when bell ringers—who often practiced ringing church bells to condition their muscles for the task—needed a quieter way to practice. They removed the bells' clappers so they remained silent as the ringers built up their strength, essentially making the bells noiseless, or "dumb."

In the *Men's Health Ultimate Dumbbell Guide,* I revealed more than 21,000 different dumbbell exercises and even explained how to create thousands of spin-off combination moves, ranging from simple to extremely complex. Those impressive numbers proved a point to anyone who ever doubted this tool's adaptability. Its compact size and uniform shape make it the easiest tool to manipulate, allowing you to rotate your wrists—or position your arms, legs, or body—in ways that can change an exercise's overall effectiveness on your muscles.

Some kettlebell and sandbag movements—particularly some of the most effective moves you can perform using either tool—require you to use both hands to handle the weight. This can limit the number of single-hand exercises, seated exercises, and other creative moves you can perform with them. But one pair of dumbbells can offer you thousands of unique options, depending on how creative you are. Here are some other upsides of this popular fitness equipment.

They're the Easiest to Master

Even the most basic kettlebell and sandbag exercises—such as the Swing and the Clean—still require a certain degree of practice before you become proficient. (Don't worry. You'll learn the proper technique quickly from this book.) However, even the most elaborate compound exercises that target multiple muscles are fairly easy to pull off with fewer mistakes with the well-designed dumbbell. That means using dumbbells can minimize your learning curve so you can start implementing a push, pull, and swing routine much sooner than you could with other tools.

They're More Muscle Specific

Many kettlebell and sandbag exercises are extremely effective at creating a better metabolic burn because they involve as many muscles as possible to push, pull, or swing the weight. But a lot of dumbbell exercises are simpler in their mechanics, giving you more options when you want to target and isolate specific muscles—particularly smaller muscle groups such as your biceps and triceps—without sharing the effort with other muscles.

They Build Strength Best

It's quite simple: The more weight you can safely handle to overload your muscles, the stronger those muscles will become. Even though kettlebells and sandbags can make you unquestionably strong, if overall strength is what you seek, dumbbells let you handle the most weight in a safer, easier-to-control manner.

The Kettlebell Edge

Although some speculate that it originated in ancient Greece, many historians believe the kettlebell (or *girya*) was first developed in the 1700s by Russian farmers, who used it as a simple tool to help measure grain and goods and as a counterweight on farm equipment. Since that time, the cast-iron weight resembling a cannonball with a thick handle has become a fitness mainstay throughout Russia. During the late 1800s to early 1900s, Ukrainian and Russian strongmen and circus performers used it to wow audiences with feats of strength.

Once kettlebells became recognized on a wider scale for their ability to combine strength training, cardiovascular fitness, and flexibility training in one workout, their popularity spread throughout the Soviet Union. In the 20th century, kettlebell lifting became the country's national sport, and the exercise tool was embraced by everyone from local athletes to Olympians and even the Red Army. In the last 2 decades, the kettlebell has finally been recognized, on a global scale, as a valuable workout tool for increasing power, endurance, stamina, strength, agility, and balance. Kettlebells tax both the cardiorespiratory and musculoskeletal systems through progressive, functional, total-body movements. Here are more key benefits of this oddly shaped resistance tool.

The Handle Has Hidden Benefits

Dumbbell and barbell bars are easy on the hands. When using them for some exercises, it's actually easy to cheat by hooking your fingers around the handle without using your thumb or by letting the weight rest more along your palms (particularly when performing certain pushing exercises, such as Shoulder or Chest Presses). But kettlebells don't allow that luxury. The handles are much thicker and a bit longer than those on typical strength training equipment, and many kettlebell exercises are quick, explosive, ballistic movements that require a tight grip of the handle at all times.

Those two differences alone force your fingers, hands, wrists, and forearms to work much harder to balance and simply manage the weight during push, pull, or swing exercises. The thick, heavy handle exercises your hand and finger muscles to build a vicelike grip that will allow you to hold heavier amounts of weight for longer periods of time when training—a side benefit that can help you achieve greater results from exercises that rely on having a stronger grip, such as Deadlifts and Rows. The more you can lift, the more lean mass you'll gain and the stronger you'll be.

Another advantage to its longer handle is hand placement. This design allows you to switch your hand position midway through an exercise so you can perform more hybrid lifts, like the Snatch and the Clean and Press. And unlike dumbbells, which are predominantly gripped at the center of the handle, a kettlebell can be gripped by the handle, by the horns (the sides of the handle), or around or underneath the ball, allowing you to alter a certain lift to make it easier or harder.

Their Shape Serves a Purpose

Although you can use kettlebells and dumbbells interchangeably for many exercises—such as Presses, Curls, and Rows—the kettlebells' odd shape affects your muscles in a slightly different way as you push, pull, or swing them.

Unlike dumbbells, which are symmetrically balanced so their weight is distributed evenly in the center of your hand, the weight of a kettlebell hangs a few inches below its handle. With the kettlebell's center of gravity shifted away from your hands, your muscles need to work harder through a greater range of motion. Depending on how you hold the kettlebell, its center of gravity actually shifts as you move through an exercise. This makes it unstable and more difficult to maneuver, which calls into action those stabilizing proprioceptive muscles mentioned earlier, as well as major muscle groups, particularly your shoulders, hamstrings, hips, lower back, and core. This is one reason why you'll notice that a kettlebell feels heavier than a dumbbell of the same weight, even if you perform the same exercises with each tool. All that extra stabilization makes your entire body work just a little bit harder than if you were using a dumbbell, which can increase the intensity of your workout.

They Strengthen the Mind-Muscle Connection

A lot of exercises that target specific muscles are so linear in movement that they take almost no thought to execute. You can actually fall into the habit of daydreaming while exercising, and you lose focus and workout intensity as a result. Kettlebells don't let that happen. Because most kettlebell exercises require a much higher level of coordination to perform, your mind is left with little choice but to concentrate and work more in tandem with your muscles. That teamwork approach also applies to complex exercises that work your upper body, lower body, and core all at once. Moving (or positioning yourself around) the kettlebell takes some concentration and a full-body effort that is dependent on all of your muscles working collectively. Unlike many dumbbell exercises that may teach certain muscles to learn to work together—such as your chest, shoulders, and triceps when doing a Chest Press—many classic kettlebell exercises require your upper body, lower body, and core to all work synergistically to push, pull, or swing the weight. Even though you don't recognize that you are using your brain to make these adjustments, you are, because the movements are complex.

They Train Muscles Men Often Forget

One of the most basic—and, by all accounts, one of the most effective—kettlebell exercises is the Swing. This simple yet complex move targets many of the muscles that guys love to ignore— the ones they can't see in the mirror.

Every time you swing the kettlebell between your legs and raise it to chest height or clean the kettlebell up to your shoulders, you're using posterior chain muscles of your body—your hamstrings, glutes, and lower back.

These "behind you" muscles are often ignored, but they're vital to total-body development, overall strength, and injury prevention, and they're vital if you want to excel at any activity that involves jumping or sprinting. If you use kettlebells, it's impossible to forget your posterior muscles because they're constantly being employed through most kettlebell exercises.

They're Way Safer Than You Think

Even though getting a kettlebell into certain positions—such as racking it by your shoulders— may initially cause the weights to brush or bang against your forearms (until you master the form), kettlebells are surprisingly safe. In fact, kettlebells require less wrist, shoulder, or upper-back flexibility than barbells or dumbbells, and they may be a smarter way to train to prevent back pain. Many traditional exercises used to work your posterior chain tend to place a higher degree of compressive force on your spine. Consider Squats and Deadlifts, for example. They can create a catch-22 situation, since the exercises meant to strengthen your back could simultaneously place your spine at a greater risk of injury. Kettlebell swings, on the other hand, can strengthen these same muscles with less compressive force and a lighter weight load, reducing your risk of injury. But the kettlebell swing is a tricky move to get right. Learn how by practicing the

Hip Hinge drill on page 104 before trying the swings beginning on page 106.

They Boost Metabolism and Burn Fat

Push, pull, or swing a kettlebell with perfect form for just 1 minute and you'll never look at other cardiovascular activities, such as running, bicycling, and stair climbing, in the same way again. Most kettlebell exercises are ballistic, high-repetition, full-body movements that affect your body in much the same way that sprinting does. It's a high-intensity pace that burns off unwanted body fat and drastically improves your cardiovascular health while simultaneously building quality muscle and boosting your overall strength by utilizing a greater percentage of fast twitch muscle fibers.

Trainers like the efficiency of kettlebell training, saying it can virtually cut your workout time in half. "Instead of lifting weights for half an hour and doing the treadmill for another half hour, you can get everything done with kettlebells in 20 minutes," said Michael Shade, kettlebell instructor at Sports Club/LA in Miami, in *ACE FitnessMatters*.

Consider this recent clinical evidence: Researchers at the University of Wisconsin–La Crosse discovered that after 8 weeks of twice weekly 20-minute workouts of alternating single-arm Snatches (intervals of 15 seconds of work and 15 seconds of rest), participants burned an average of 400 calories. "They were burning at least 20.2 calories per minute, which is off the charts," said lead researcher John Porcari, PhD. "That's equivalent to running a

6-minute mile pace" or cross-country skiing uphill at a fast pace.

Total-body workouts like the kettlebell Snatch routine can provide much higher-intensity workouts than a standard weight-training routine. Heart rate data from that University of Wisconsin–La Crosse study, which was sponsored by the American Council on Exercise (ACE), demonstrated just how intense kettlebell workouts can be. The average heart rate during the kettlebell Snatch workout was 93 percent of the kettlebell HR max for all subjects. "But some people averaged, for the 20-minute workout, 99 percent of heart rate max," said Porcari. "Anytime you're using that much muscle effort, it's going to be a vigorous workout."

Another point that makes kettlebells potentially a better fat-loss friend is how joint friendly they are. Running, cycling, and other high-intensity aerobic activities typically place stress on your knees and joints. To make matters worse, these same activities typically work one side of your body while neglecting the other—running, for example, primarily works the muscles behind you (lower back, hamstrings, and glutes) but not the muscles in front of you (quadriceps and abdominals). Over time, this can allow stronger muscles on one side of your body to overpower weaker muscles, causing a muscular imbalance that can increase your risk of injury and lead to posture and joint issues.

The Sandbag Edge

The invention of the sandbag may predate both dumbbells and kettlebells, but experts seem to find its origins harder to lock down than the other two. The reason is obvious: Unlike dumbbells and kettlebells (tools created for the sole purpose of building strength, power, and coordination), people have been putting stuff in sacks and hauling them around for centuries. Whether it was to trade and store a product like flour, sugar, or rice; to fortify military positions; or to act as a means of flood control, animal skins or other bags filled with some heavy, shifting substance have been building muscle on men for as long as men have been shouldering stuff in sacks. That said, sandbags have been commonly used by athletes (primarily wrestlers) for a few hundred years. In the early 1900s, they gained popularity among strongmen as a means of both building and displaying their strength. These awkward objects soon became favored by other types of athletes and soldiers who were either participating in combat sports or looking for a training tool that mimicked the dead weight and unstable resistance of an opponent. In the recent wars in Iraq and Afghanistan, marines used the sandbags fortifying their bunkers as tools to keep their muscles in shape. As these soldiers know, there are many reasons to make sandbags a part of your workout gear.

They're the Least Expensive Solution

Your body doesn't care how much money you blew on a piece of exercise equipment. All that matters to your muscles is getting a great workout. You can't buy a cheaper fitness tool than the one with a name that describes the only two materials you need to make it: sand and a bag.

Even though there are pricy sandbags on the market—ones with convenient straps and other features built in that can make maneuvering the sandbag easier—it only takes an investment of a few dollars to make your own sandbag. Even the most basic sandbag, which you'll learn how to make in the next chapter, will allow you to perform sandbag exercises just as effectively as a higher-end product.

They Develop a Bone-Grinding Handshake

Although dumbbells require a strong grip during certain movements and kettlebells demand a constant grip throughout most movements, your hands and fingers get a break at certain moments, especially once these weights are positioned where they need to be.

But with a sandbag, your hands and fingers must work constantly to pull off most exercises. You may even find yourself constantly gripping and regripping the bag just to maintain control as you push, pull, or swing it—an inconvenience that can dynamically boost your grip strength.

Workouts Are Never the Same Twice

Because the sandbag has a shifting center of mass that constantly changes as you raise and lower it, your body has to adjust to manage and stabilize its ever-changing shape. That makes each and every repetition—no matter whether you're pushing, pulling, or swinging the sandbag—slightly different than the previous one. All of that extra muscle recruitment means that your body has to use more energy as you exercise, which could potentially help you burn additional calories and blast extra fat.

They Build Strength You Can Use

Think about the last heavy thing you had to pick up and move—a bag of water softener salt, an old refrigerator you were throwing out, or your 5-year-old nephew. Was the heavy object perfectly balanced? Did it have convenient handles for gripping? When it comes to developing functional strength and power, neither a dumbbell nor a kettlebell beats a sandbag. Many of the push, pull, and swing exercises for sandbags genuinely mimic real life movements and lifts that the average guy makes every day. Pick up a heavy garbage bag, lift your kid out of a car seat, toss a suitcase into the overhead bin—those are all movements you can mimic with a sandbag.

They're Unconventional

Because of its unique features—particularly its conforming shape and lack of heavy metal—a sandbag is ideal for replicating a range of push, pull, and swing exercises that are either impossible, or simply not safe, to do with dumbbells or kettlebells (or most other traditional strength training equipment, for that matter).

You can flip it and throw it without worrying about needing to repair drywall. You can drop it in your garage without cracking the concrete or drag it across the hardwood floor with nary a scratch. And because a sandbag is pliable, it's able to conform to your body when placed across your shoulders or against your chest. That makes it an ideal training tool for experimenting with a range of unconventional brute strength and intense endurance drills, such as Bear Hug Squats, dragging and tossing exercises, Shouldering (pulling the sandbag from the floor onto your shoulder), and weighted sprints, just to name a few.

They're the Most Travel Friendly

Even though sandbags may take up the most space when filled, they generally take up the least amount of space—and weigh the least—when empty. That makes a sandbag the smartest play of the three if you plan to take your push, pull, and swing routine on the road. All it takes is investing in some sand once you reach your destination, and sand averages $3 to $4 for 50 pounds at any hardware store. Or better yet, it's absolutely free if you're travelling somewhere near a beach. (*Psst*—remember to practice leave-no-trace lifting: Put back the sand before you leave the beach.)

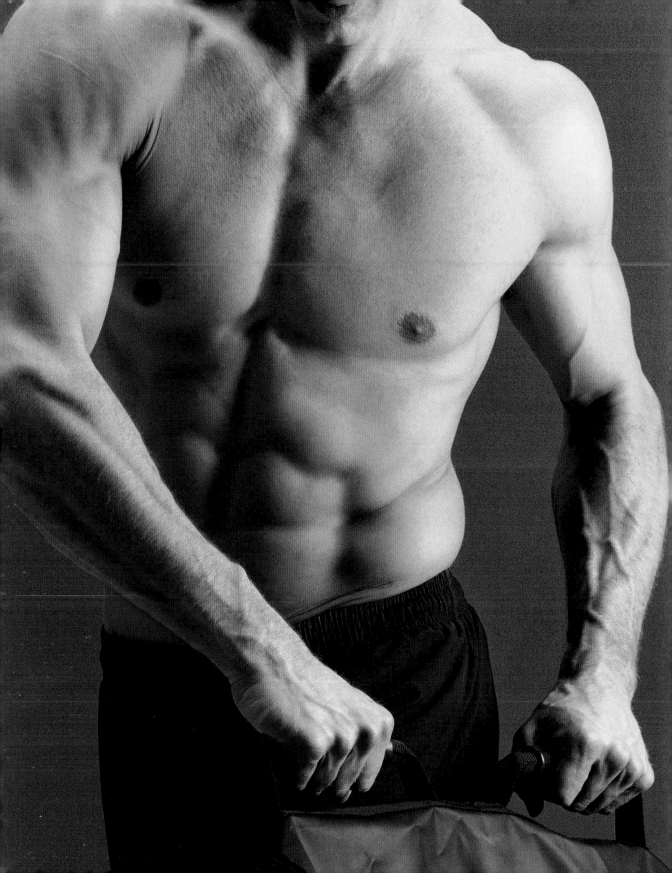

CHAPTER 3

OLD-SCHOOL TOOLS

WHAT YOU NEED TO SUCCEED

You can't begin to push, pull, and swing unless you have the right stuff to push, pull, and swing. This chapter is about your choices.

Of course, you could go outside and pick up a large, heavy rock to use for most of the exercises in this book. But you'd be better off getting yourself dumbbells, kettlebells, or a sandbag.

Note the word *or*. To use this book, you only need one type of gear: a set of dumbbells, the right size kettlebell, or a sandbag. Heck, you can even make an excellent sandbag easily at home, and we give you instructions for doing so on page 24. The point is, you don't have to spend a lot of cash gearing up to reap the benefits of the Push, Pull, Swing philosophy.

The power of this book lies in the fact that you can use any of these tools to achieve the results you want. But you also can incorporate *all three* pieces of equipment for your workouts, if you are so inclined. Each offers unique advantages for total-body muscle growth and fitness. As you advance in your weight training, you may find that you want to add all three pieces of equipment to your arsenal of workout gear. It's up to you.

Dumbbells

There are three types of dumbbells on the market, but which type you choose to invest in depends entirely on what works best for you.

FIXED-WEIGHT. This style of dumbbell—typically the type found in health clubs and gyms—is one solid piece of metal that weighs a certain amount. Although you'll find them made from a range of materials, from inexpensive cast iron to high-priced polished chrome, your muscles will get the same workout no matter how large a hit your wallet takes. Typically, these dumbbells are hexagonal.

PLATE-LOADED ADJUSTABLE. This type of dumbbell—basically a small, 12- to 15-inch bar that holds standard weight plates—works much like a barbell, giving you the ability to add or remove weight plates on either end.

You can buy them in standard sizes of 10, 20, 25 pounds, etc. However, you can also choose to create your own by purchasing a pair of standard handles, plates, and collars for the ends. (Depending on the type you buy, the collars clamp, thread onto, or pinch the bar to keep the weight from sliding off.)

SELECTORIZED ADJUSTABLE. This advanced type of dumbbell—which has only been available since the early 1990s—allows you to quickly choose the amount of weight you want to load onto the bar and lets you change the weight without removing or reattaching collars.

Most use a series of thin, interconnecting weight plates that sit inside a special base. Before you lift the dumbbell from its base, you turn a knob, press a button, or move a lever to select how heavy you want the dumbbell to be. The correct number of plates mechanically attaches to the handle, leaving the remaining plates inside the base. Most brands of selectorized dumbbells allow you to change the weight in 5-pound increments.

Picking the Perfect Pair of Dumbbells

IF YOU HAVE THE SPACE AND BUDGET, FIXED-WEIGHT DUMBBELLS ARE YOUR BEST BET. The convenience of being able to grab them and start pushing, pulling, or swinging them instantly is the reason they're the dumbbell style of choice in gyms worldwide.

But before you buy, remember this: Because they're unchangeable (unlike the other two types), you may have little choice but to shell out a lot of money for a variety of sizes in order to perform exercises that require lighter or heavier weight loads. One bonus of fixed-weight dumbbells is that most of them have hexagonal-shaped heads, so they won't roll on uneven floors like plate-loaded dumbbells will. And because they won't roll, hex dumbbells are great for doing exercises such as Neutral-Grip Pushups and T-Raises.

IF YOU HAVE TO MAKE ENDS MEET, STICK WITH PLATE-LOADED DUMBBELLS. If you don't mind constantly fumbling with collars and weight plates between exercises, one pair of adjustable dumbbells with enough weight plates can be cheaper than having to buy various sizes of fixed-weight dumbbells.

But before you buy, remember this: Using an adjustable dumbbell when lifting heavy weights can sometimes be a bit cumbersome. Unlike fixed-weight dumbbells, which are more compact, plate-loaded dumbbells will be as large as their heaviest plates, which tend to be larger than lighter-weight plates. This can make certain exercises more difficult to do comfortably.

IF YOU HAVE THE MONEY, INVEST IN A PAIR OF SELECTORIZED ADJUSTABLE DUMBBELLS. Although most high-end, high-weight versions start in the hundreds of dollars and can easily run you over a thousand dollars, the ability to create dozens of different pairs of dumbbells (ranging from as little as 2.5 pounds up to 175 pounds per dumbbell), all from a piece of equipment that takes up the space of a small nightstand, is hard to beat.

But before you buy, remember this: Even if money is no option, some selectorized adjustable dumbbells aren't as easy to use as others. With some brands, you may find yourself fighting with the mechanics of the dumbbell, which can waste valuable time if you're following a routine that has you resting for less time between sets.

Another issue some lifters have with these dumbbells is the extra lifting they have to do in order to change the weight between exercises. Having to lift each dumbbell back into its base after every exercise just to change the weight may not seem like a hassle now, but wait until you have to change it after performing exercises such as heavy Deadlifts, Bent-Over Rows, and other multijoint compound exercises. Because your muscles need to utilize the time between sets to get a thorough amount of rest,

having to hoist each dumbbell back into its base can minimize that valuable recovery time and hurt the rest of your workout.

WHERE TO BUY: You can get great deals on used fixed-weight and plate-loaded dumbbells at garage sales and through Craigslist.org. Most large retailers carry them new. Popular brands of selectorized adjustable dumbbells include Bowflex, PowerBlock, and Universal.

Kettlebells

Because of their Russian heritage, kettlebells are measured in kilograms (kg), instead of pounds (lb). And unlike dumbbells (which increase by 1-, 2½-, and 5-pound increments) and sandbags (which you can adjust to practically any poundage you wish, down to the ounce), kettlebells take far greater leaps from one size to the next. They also offer fewer size choices.

Decades ago, you would have been hard-pressed to find more than three different sizes—with 16 kg, 24 kg, and 32 kg being the most common. Today, the most common sizes you're likely to find are:

▶ 4 kg (8.8 lb)
▶ 8 kg (17.6 lb)
▶ 10 kg (22 lb)
▶ 12 kg (26.5 lb)
▶ 14 kg (30.8 lb)
▶ 16 kg (35.3 lb)
▶ 18 kg (39.7 lb)
▶ 20 kg (44.1 lb)
▶ 22 kg (48.5 lb)

▶ 24 kg (52.9 lb)
▶ 26 kg (57.3 lb)
▶ 28 kg (61.7 lb)
▶ 32 kg (70.5 lb)
▶ 36 kg (79.4 lb)
▶ 40 kg (88.2 lb)
▶ 44 kg (97 lb)
▶ 48 kg (105.8 lb)

Picking the Perfect Kettlebell

So which one is just right for you?

Most experts feel that the best size for men to start with is a 16-kg (or 35-lb) kettlebell. One easy way to determine if a 16-kg size is either too heavy or too light for your body is to try to push it over your head with one arm and lock your elbow. You should be able to keep the weight stable but still experience a certain degree of resistance. If you can't muster the strength to keep it there for 10 seconds, choose a lighter weight.

Just don't make the mistake of going too light. Many kettlebell exercises—especially many of the mainstay moves, such as Swings and Cleans—are a lot easier to learn using a weight that offers your body a challenging level of resistance.

The same warning can be said about choosing a size that's too heavy, which can make it much harder to learn proper form. To be honest, if you're stronger than the average guy, you may be able to handle a size that's heavier (between 18 and 24 kg). But if you're new to kettlebell training, it may pay off in the long run to start with an average-size kettlebell so that you can focus on form.

Once you feel comfortable with your choice, you're done—for now, at least. Most fitness

KICK THE TIRES, BUT WATCH YOUR TOES

You may think that it's hard to screw up manufacturing a big round ball of metal with a handle on it, but as kettlebells have risen in popularity over the last 2 decades, so have the number of companies churning out a variety of different versions of this classic exercise tool. Making sure you're investing in a quality kettlebell is critical, especially because among the push, pull, and swing trio, it's the tool that could potentially do the most damage if it breaks midworkout. To make sure you're not going to need a contractor down the road, here are a few things you should do when purchasing a kettlebell.

SKIP THE SHINY STUFF. You want to invest in a kettlebell that's not coated with any material, such as vinyl covers or a nonskid base. Although a colorful, coated one may look nicer, the biggest issue is that it may not allow you to see the kettlebell's construction. Buying a plain cast-iron one allows you to see whether the bell is made from one solid piece. Cheaper versions sometimes forge the ball and handle separately and then connect them—increasing your risk of having the ball break off down the road.

GRAB THE HANDLE WITH BOTH HANDS. The handle should be large enough so that both hands fit comfortably without touching each other.

GRAB THE HANDLE WITH ONE HAND. You want to be sure that the tips of your fingers don't touch your palm when they're wrapped around the handle. If the handle is too thin, it can make certain exercises (such as Renegade Rows) harder on your hands and wrists, particularly when you're doing Snatches and Cleans. If the handle is too thick for your hand, it can be dangerous to use.

ASK FOR AT LEAST A 1-YEAR GUARANTEE. If a company says no, chances are there's a reason for it.

WHERE TO BUY: Most large sporting goods stores (like Dick's Sporting Goods) and big box stores (like Walmart) now carry kettlebells. Online, performbetter.com carries quality kettlebells.

experts recommend that people learn proper technique first, particularly with the Clean and Press, Snatch, Squat, and Swing. But even once you've mastered these four moves, you may want to wait before investing in a heavier kettlebell. The smarter purchase would be a second bell of the same size, which would allow you to pull off a variety of more advanced double kettlebell exercises, where you hold a bell in each hand rather than having both hands hold a single kettlebell.

There are also certain dumbbell exercises that can be mimicked with the kettlebell, but they're not as easily pulled off if you have only one. As you go through this book and begin to select some of the exercises you believe work best for your fitness goals, keep in mind that you may need to invest in a few pairs of kettlebells in various sizes.

Sandbags

When it comes to this final push, pull, and swing tool, you have two choices: make a purchase, or make your own. A lot of guys start with homemade versions and then progress to a commercial sandbag once they become hooked on sandbag training. I'll cover both types in this chapter.

Picking the Perfect Sandbag

With the popularity of sandbags on the rise, more and more products have entered the market. Some can run you as high as hundreds of dollars and come with instructional DVDs. Here's what to look for.

MAKE SURE IT CAN TAKE A BEATING—BUT THAT YOUR HANDS WON'T. If you can test it in person, put it through its paces. A sandbag that seems like it's going to leak most likely will.

You want to look for a sandbag made from a heavy-duty material such as canvas—something that feels impossible to puncture. But more importantly, take the time to rub and roll your fists along the bag. It doesn't have to be baby smooth, but it shouldn't tear up your hands, either. Some cheaper models use materials that may be indestructible, but they can feel like sandpaper on your skin, bringing your routine to a halt before your muscles get a thorough workout.

HAVE SAND AT THE READY. Ironically, most sandbags don't come preloaded with sand (or any high-density material, for that matter) because of how inefficient it would be to ship them. Do yourself the favor of getting your sand before you buy your bag. Some lifters prefer to use dry rice because it weighs less. It's your call.

The reason: The moment you get your sandbag, you should immediately fill it to its capacity (even if you're not strong enough yet to use it at that level) and try picking it up and swinging it from every handle. You want to be sure every strap and every seam is as well constructed as it should be.

ASK ABOUT THE RETURN POLICY. Compared to the other two pieces of equipment, sandbags are not only the easiest to break or rip—blame that whole cast iron versus canvas thing—but they are also the most likely to take a major beating, since some sandbag drills may require you to drag the bag across the floor or toss it onto the pavement or dirt. Knowing the

THE SANDBOX:
HOW TO MAKE YOUR OWN GEAR

Making a homegrown workout sandbag is as easy as tossing a few shovelfuls of beach sand into an old canvas daypack. But you'll want something sturdier that won't get you jailed for stealing public sand. Here's how to make sandbags that can weather tough workouts.

What You'll Need

- Several contractor-grade, heavy-duty plastic trash bags
- A few bags of playground sand (it typically comes in 50-pound bags) or rice
- Roll of duct tape
- 2 sturdy canvas duffel bags (get a few different sizes if you plan to make several sandbags of different weights) or old backpacks
- Bathroom scale
- Shovel or a large plastic cup
- Scissors

Build It

1 Grab your scale, place an empty heavy-duty trash bag on top of it, and fill it until you've reached your desired weight. (Some lifters prefer rice over sand because it's lighter and isn't as prone to spilling.) For men, between 30 and 70 pounds is a great starting point. If you're making sandbags of various sizes, write the weight of each sandbag on a piece of duct tape and stick it to the bag. Note: You can choose to make one large, sand-filled garbage bag with the weight you plan to use or make several smaller bags of various weights that you can switch around to change the weight of your sandbag.

2 Twist the top of the sand-filled trash bag a few times, but leave enough space in the bag so that the sand can move around inside it. (If you don't, the sandbag will feel stiffer, more predictable, and more stable when you eventually use it.) Seal the bag tightly with duct tape.

3 Place your sand-filled bag inside one or two more trash bags, sealing each one securely with duct tape.

4 Place the sand-filled bags in your duffel, zip it shut, and you're ready to go.

5 If you're still paranoid about sand spillage, you can take the extra step of duct taping the zipper. However, keep in mind that tape on the outside of the bag may make it more difficult to grab at certain places, and it will make changing the weight of the bag (if you plan to use several smaller bags and change the weight for different exercises) more time-consuming.

HOME GROWN: Use old duffels, backpacks, heavy-duty trash bags or zipper-lock bags, sand or rice, duct tape, and a scale.

rules on replacement if it tears after an intense workout may be the deciding factor when you're choosing between several different sandbags.

REMEMBER WHY YOU'RE BUYING ONE IN THE FIRST PLACE. One of the things that makes sandbags so unique compared to dumbbells and kettlebells is how they force you to dig into the bag with your fingers to get a firm grip—and then constantly maintain that tight grip in order to use them. Some purists feel that the newer designs offer too many handholds all over the bags (such as handles and straps) that defeat the purpose of training with a sandbag by minimizing the extra grip and stability benefits they naturally offer.

Personally, I like sandbags with straps or handles because they are more versatile. The straps make it easier to mimic many dumbbell and kettlebell exercises. But just because they are built in doesn't mean you have to use them all the time. A good piece of equipment allows you to exercise the way you wish to exercise.

WHERE TO BUY: You can buy burlap bags, heavy-duty plastic bags, and playground sand at any hardware or garden store to make your own (see opposite). If you want a bag specifically designed with handles for exercise, some good bags include Rogue Fitness bags (roguefitness .com) and the Ultimate Sandbag Training System (ultimatesandbagtraining.com). There are even hybrid sandbags that are essentially a cross between a sandbag, dumbbell, and kettlebell. Search for Sandbells at performbetter.com.

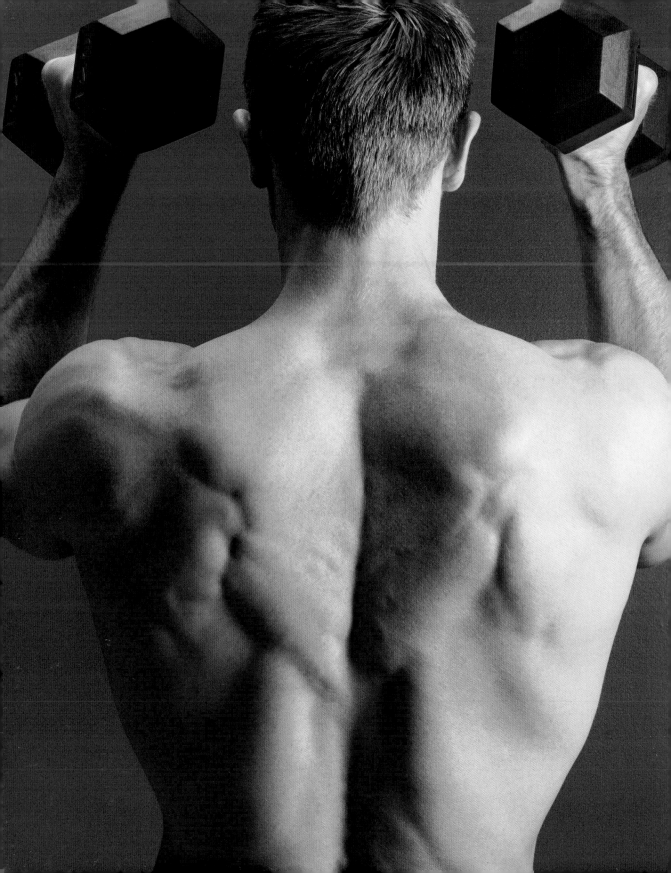

CHAPTER 4

YOUR MUSCLES AND HOW THEY MOVE

THE ANATOMY OF PUSH, PULL, AND SWING

"Leave no stone unturned" is the perfect idiom for how we should approach building strong, symmetrical muscles. We should ignore no muscles, no matter how small, to achieve true total-body fitness for optimal functioning in the real world. But to do that properly, one needs to be familiar with all of those "stones."

The mission of the push, pull, swing concept is to ensure that you engage all of your muscles, not just the ones that look good in a mirror, during your workouts. Therefore, it pays to get to know the muscles that you're looking to improve. Pushing, pulling, and swinging movements often engage more than one muscle group at a time, so this guide will also give you a better understanding of how they work together.

The Muscles That Help Push

Chest (Pectorals)

You actually have two separate groups of muscles that make up your chest. The larger of the two is the pectoralis major, the top layer that lies closest to your skin. The fibers of this muscle originate at three locations: your collarbone, your breastbone, and your ribs just below your breastbone. From there, the fibers stretch across both sides of your chest in a fan shape, starting wide at the center of your body and tapering together at the sides of your body to attach to the top of your humerus (upper arm bone).

The smaller of the two muscle groups is the pectoralis minor, which rests underneath your pectoralis major. This thinner, more triangular muscle starts at your third, fourth, and fifth ribs and attaches near your shoulder joint.

HOW THEY WORK: Together, both muscles are responsible for moving your upper arms toward the center of your body and assist with drawing your shoulders forward. Whenever you either push a weight above your chest or push your body away from a stationary object (like the floor, when performing a Pushup), your pectorals shorten in order to pull your arms across your chest and bring them together.

Triceps Brachii

Located along the backs of your upper arms, your triceps are composed of three separate muscles, or heads: the lateral head, the medial head, and the long head. The three heads each start at one of two locations—your upper arm bone or your shoulder blade—then come together at your forearm, attaching to a tendon that connects to your elbow bone.

HOW THEY WORK: All three heads work together to extend your elbows, which is what you're doing every time you straighten your arm from a bent position. This happens whenever you push a weight over your head or above your chest, for example. However, your triceps brachii also help out with other jobs, which include stabilizing your shoulder joints during certain pushing movements and aiding your upper back muscles with arm adduction (which happens when you bring your arms down and back toward your body).

Quadriceps

Your quads—the muscles that rest along the fronts of your thighs—divide into four separate heads: the vastus intermedius, the rectus femoris, the vastus lateralis, and the vastus medialis. The vastus intermedius attaches to and covers much of the front and sides of your femur (your thighbone) but is not visible, as it lies below the rectus femoris. The rectus femoris starts at your pelvis and runs down your thigh in front of the vastus intermedius. The vastus lateralis and medialis begin at the back of your femur laterally and medially, respectively. All four muscles run down your thigh and converge at the patellar tendon, which attaches along the upper part of your tibia (shinbone).

HOW THEY WORK: Your quadriceps are mainly responsible for extending your knees (straightening your legs), but they also help to support and stabilize your knee joints, particularly the inner and outer sides. Because many of the pushing exercises that target your quadriceps also involve your lower legs, your quads often work in unison with your calves.

Calves

Along the backs of your lower legs are two sets of muscle groups: the gastrocnemius and the soleus. The gastrocnemius (the larger of the two) is the one you can see. The soleus is hidden underneath the gastrocnemius and attaches just below your knee and at your Achilles tendon. Together, both sets of muscles combine to form the diamond-shaped muscle that extends from the back of your knee to your ankle.

HOW THEY WORK: The gastrocnemius's job is to flex your foot, which is what you do whenever you elevate your heels. The soleus does the exact same thing, but only when your knees are bent.

The Muscles That Help Pull
Trapezius and Rhomboids

Considered part of your upper back, the trapezius is a flat, triangle-shaped muscle that begins at the base of your skull and attaches itself to the back of your collarbone and shoulder blades. Underneath your trapezius are your rhomboids, which are positioned in the middle of your upper back, right between your shoulder blades.

HOW THEY WORK: Your trapezius is responsible for scapular elevation (when you shrug your arms up), scapular depression (when you pull your shoulder blades down), and scapular adduction (when you pull your shoulder blades together). Your rhomboids also

help out your trapezius whenever you pull your shoulder blades toward each other.

Latissimus Dorsi

Your lats—the largest muscles of your back—are a set of fan-shaped muscles that start low on your spine, spread across the width of your back, and taper off at your upper arm bones (where they meet your shoulders).

HOW THEY WORK: Their primary role is to pull your arms from a raised position back down to your sides. Also, whenever your arms are extended in front of your torso, your lats are responsible for pulling your arms down toward your torso.

However, they also help stabilize your torso during other exercises (particularly moves that target your arms, such as Biceps Curls), and they help to rotate your upper arm internally, which plays a big part in giving you that extra snap of power whenever you punch or throw. Each of these jobs gets a little help from the teres major—a smaller muscle that runs from the outer edge of the scapula to the humerus.

Biceps Brachii

This muscle is located in the front of your upper arm and is made up of two separate heads that each attach at your shoulder socket and insert onto your radius—one of the two bones of your forearm. Wedged between your biceps and upper arm bone is the brachialis, a thin muscle that attaches to your ulna—the other bone of your forearm.

HOW THEY WORK: Your biceps are responsible for elbow flexion (when you bend your arm at the elbow) to draw your lower arms toward your shoulders. They also rotate your lower arms from side to side (known as supination) to turn your palms from an up position to a down position and vice versa. Your brachialis also helps move your lower arms toward your shoulders, but only when your palms are either facing down or in toward your body.

Forearms

The real estate between your elbows and your hands—otherwise known as your forearms—contains two sets of muscles: your wrist extensors and your wrist flexors. If you want your arms to look bigger, pay attention to your forearms.

HOW THEY WORK: Your wrist extensors are located on the outside of your forearm, and they allow you to bend (or pull) your wrists backward. Your wrist flexors are found along the inside of your forearm, and they allow you to curl (or pull) your wrists forward.

Hamstrings

Your hamstrings are made up of three separate muscles comprising the entire back of your thigh—the biceps femoris (found on the outer rear portion of your thigh) and the semitendinosus and semimembranosus (the two muscles that make up the bulk of your inner rear thigh). Each attaches at your pelvic bone, runs down the back of your thigh, then connects to either your shinbone or the head of your fibula.

HOW THEY WORK: Individually, these three muscles help turn your knees inward and turn your feet outward. But when united, they collectively flex (or bend) your knees and extend your hips (kick your legs back behind you). However, they don't work alone—other muscles, including your hip flexors, glutes, and erector spinae muscles, help out as well.

The Muscles That Help Push and Pull at the Same Time

Deltoids

The muscles you confidently hang your coat over are actually divided into three heads—your anterior deltoids (located in the front of your shoulders), your medial deltoids (located along the sides), and your posterior deltoids (located behind your shoulders).

The anterior and medial deltoids start at your collarbone, while the posterior deltoids start on your scapula (your shoulder blade). All three heads come together and attach themselves to your humerus (upper arm bone).

HOW THEY WORK: Collectively, all three parts of your deltoids are responsible for moving your arms away from your torso, even though each performs a different task. Your anterior deltoids raise your arms up in front of you, your medial deltoids lift your arms up and out to your sides, and your posterior deltoids raise your arms up and behind your body.

The three heads also act as secondary movers during many pushing and pulling exercises. Your anterior deltoids assist your pectoral muscles in many pushing exercises that strengthen your chest, while your posterior deltoids assist in many pulling exercises that involve your teres major (upper back), trapezius, and rhomboid muscles.

Gluteals

You have three separate muscles to thank if you've ever been complemented on your backside. Your gluteus maximus—one of the largest and strongest muscles in your body—is responsible for creating the rounded shape of your rear end. It originates at your pelvic bone and ends along the back of your thighbone. Your gluteus medius and gluteus minimus start and end in the same two places, but they rest directly below your gluteus maximus, along the outside of your hips.

HOW THEY WORK: Your gluteus maximus's main job is hip extension, which is what happens whenever you draw your leg back behind you. It

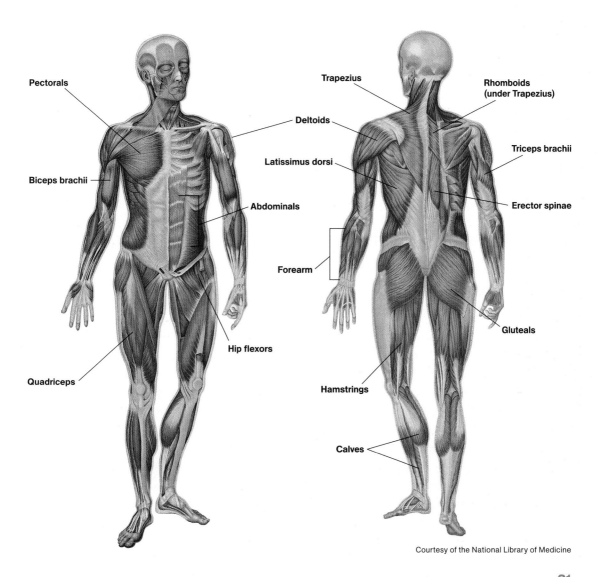

Pectorals

Biceps brachii

Deltoids

Latissimus dorsi

Abdominals

Forearm

Hip flexors

Quadriceps

Trapezius

Rhomboids
(under Trapezius)

Triceps brachii

Erector spinae

Gluteals

Hamstrings

Calves

Courtesy of the National Library of Medicine

also helps your body stand up from a squatting position by straightening your hips. Meanwhile, your gluteus medius and minimus work together to extend your leg out to the side, rotate your thigh inward when your hip is bent, and rotate your thigh outward when your leg is straight.

Although many hip-dominant pulling exercises that train your hamstrings (such as Deadlifts, Straight Leg Deadlifts, and Swings) target your glutes simultaneously, all three muscles are also activated and assist when performing quad dominant pushing exercises for your legs, such as Squats and Lunges.

The Muscles That Help Swing

Your midsection or core is made up of more than two dozen muscles that stabilize your spine, as well as bend your torso forward, backward, from side to side, and—in the case of any swinging exercise—rotate it in every possible direction. Here are these critical muscles, in no particular order.

Abdominals

Your abdominals are comprised of four muscle groups. Your rectus abdominis—the long sheet of muscle in front—isn't just responsible for giving you that six-pack look, but also for pulling your torso toward your hips. Its other, equally important job is to act as a counterbalance against the muscles that extend your spine so that your posture is perfect.

The next two muscles are your obliques—your external obliques, which run diagonally down from your lower ribs to the front top of your pelvis and pubic bone, and your internal obliques, which are found underneath, running diagonally to your external obliques. Together, their main jobs are rotating your torso and lateral flexion (bending your torso in toward your hips).

The final of the four is your transverse abdominis. Running deep beneath your obliques, this thin muscle layer, which stretches from your lower ribs to your pubic bone, pulls your abdominal wall inward. This protects your internal organs while helping to support your spine.

HOW THEY WORK: Together, all four support and assist in moving your torso through various planes of motion—bending your body from side to side, twisting right and left, and lowering and raising your torso. *Note:* When talking about the "core," I'm including the muscles of the lower back, which work together with the abdominals to support the spine.

Lower Back

Although the muscles that make up your lower back are many, the major group that men focus on is the erector spinae, or spinal erectors. These deep muscles rest along both sides of your spinal column, starting at the back of your skull and attaching to your pelvis.

HOW THEY WORK: With the help of other smaller muscles, both erectors extend your spine—straightening it after it's been flexed forward—as well as bend your spine posteriorly (arch your back). They are also responsible for helping to support your spinal column all day long.

Hip Flexors

Located along the fronts of your thighs, your hip flexors are actually divided primarily into two muscle groups: the iliacus (which starts at your pelvis and attaches to your thighbone) and the psoas major (which originates on your lumbar vertebrae and also connects to your thighbone).

HOW THEY WORK: Their main task is to pull your thighs toward your midsection. When you're standing, it's these muscles that help raise your thighs up, but when you're lying flat, it's these same muscles that also lift your legs toward your torso or lift your torso into a Situp position.

That's an overview of the major muscles and muscle groups involved in every push, pull, and swing movement. But that's hardly all of the muscles that contribute to moving in all three planes. By incorporating pushing, pulling, and swinging movements into your workouts, you'll have the best chance of activating the greatest number of muscles—both large and small—for true, total-body strength, muscle tone, and endurance.

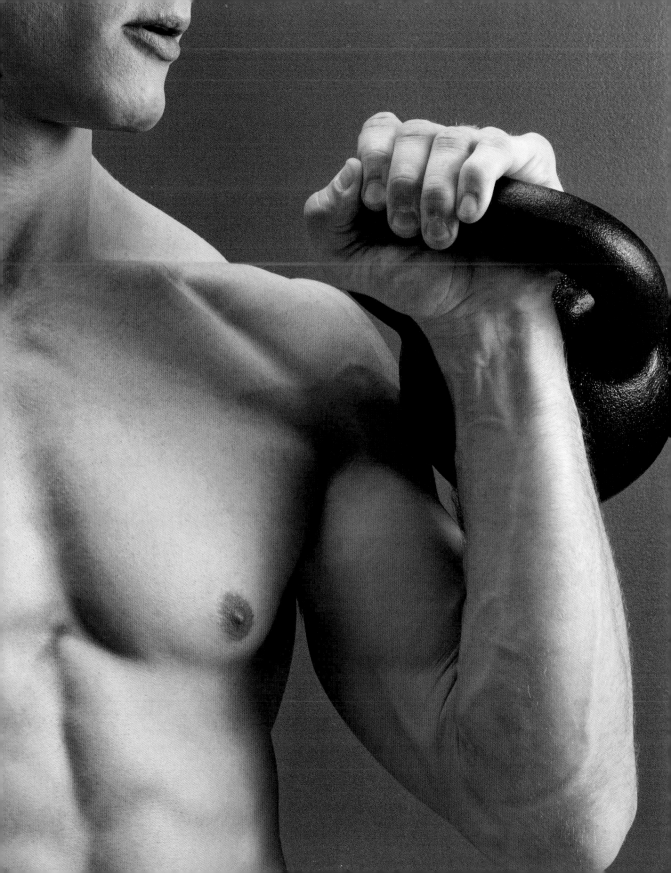

CHAPTER 5

NUTRITION TO POWER YOUR WORKOUTS

SIX STEPS FOR EATING RIGHT WHILE TRAINING FOR A LEANER, MORE MUSCULAR BODY

I despise the word *diet*. People associate it with losing weight, but that's not all that a diet can do. By definition, "diet" means the kind and amount of food prescribed for a person for a special reason. After all, some skinny guys want to put on weight. Others aren't concerned at all with packing on muscle or shedding love handles. Instead, they want to become stronger or faster or better at their sport. Still others want to peel back the years

and see the body they remember having in their twenties.

This isn't a diet book with a specific goal in mind. But that doesn't mean a smart nutrition strategy isn't just as important as that dumbbell, kettlebell, and sandbag you're moving around. It is. To get the most out of any of the Push, Pull, Swing exercises and workouts in this book, you have to eat right to fuel the muscle repair and building process that's so critical to all of those common goals, from weight loss and strength building to sports performance and good overall health. Team up your workouts with a fueling system built around these six important steps.

Step #1: Figure Out How Much Fuel You Need

Deciding how many calories you need to eat each day may sound complicated, but it's far easier than most people realize. Most experts agree that the best approach is to eat for your target body weight. Whether you want to lose weight or gain weight, that magic number that you want to see on the scale takes a certain number of calories each day to maintain. That number is how many calories you should be eating.

The fastest way to come up with that number is with this formula: First decide how much you want to weigh, then multiply that number by 10 to 12, based on your goal and activity level. If your goal is to lose weight and you exercise once or twice a week, use 10 as your multiplier. If you are exercising more often, you'll need more energy, so you should multiply by 12. The product of those numbers is the total calories you should be devouring for the day. For example, if you currently weigh 195 pounds, but you want to weigh 175 pounds and you are doing these Push, Pull, Swing workouts 4 or 5 days a week, then you would multiply 175 x 12. For you, 2,100 calories would be the right number of calories to eat each day.

The right multiplier really depends on how active you are. So, if you are also playing basketball or doing other calorie-burning activities in addition to your Push, Pull, Swing strength training, you'll want to multiply the weight you wish to be by maybe 14, instead of 12. If you are doing a lot of high-volume workouts and you wish to gain muscle weight, you can increase your calorie intake up to 16 calories per pound. Just be sure to consume enough protein, as described later.

Step #2: Divide That Number by 7

Why 7? Because that's how many meals you're going to be eating throughout the course of your day. Increasing your meal frequency increases the amount of fat you burn for energy and stabilizes your insulin levels, which means your body doesn't store as many excess calories as fat. But what most men forget is that their bodies burn calories consuming, digesting, and metabolizing each meal. Roughly 10 percent of the calories you burn each day is spent on what is known as the thermic effect of feeding, so the more you eat, the more often your metabolism gets stoked during the day so you can break down every bite.

By splitting up your daily calories into seven smaller, more frequent portions (all roughly equal in size), you'll help keep fat at bay while allowing your body to get the nutrients and protein it needs to build lean muscle. Your best bet: Divide your daily calorie allowance into seven smaller meals—breakfast, lunch, and dinner, with four snacks: one right before breakfast, one between breakfast and lunch, one between lunch and dinner, and a final snack right before you go to sleep.

YOUR PRE- AND POSTWORKOUT EATING PLAN

What you eat before and after each workout can have a huge effect on the results you can expect to see after weeks of pushing, pulling, and swinging. Follow these rules and you'll always have enough energy to get the most from every workout and enough nutrients to help you put on—and protect—new muscle.

To make sure you have enough energy to push yourself, experts recommend eating a simple meal with at least 200 calories, 20 grams of protein, and 30 grams of carbohydrates an hour before you work out. Some good options to try: a small protein shake with some berries mixed in, a tall glass of chocolate milk, a piece of chicken breast and a small apple, or a small sandwich made with 4 ounces of deli turkey and a slice of American cheese on whole wheat bread.

When your workout is over, the real workout starts taking place within your body as your freshly beaten-down muscles begin to repair themselves. By consuming protein (between 20 and 30 grams) as quickly as possible afterward, you'll give your body what it needs to rebuild muscle. The fastest way to get your muscles what they need is by mixing one scoop of whey protein powder with water.

You also want to eat some form of fast-acting, easily digestible carbohydrate, like a slice of white bread, some instant rice, or a banana, for example. This trick will help you restore any lost glycogen—the stored glucose your body uses for immediate energy—but it will also cause your body to release insulin, a hormone that is believed to help repair muscles faster by enhancing protein synthesis.

Step #3: Know the Right Ratios

Each of the main three macronutrients—protein, carbohydrates, and fats—serves a different role, which is why each affects your body in a different way and is needed in a different amount. Having the right mix of each will ensure that your body has enough protein to build muscle, while providing you with an even stream of energy that won't drastically ebb and flow, which can cause your body to store more of the calories you're eating as unwanted body fat.

Protein

Eat 1 gram for every pound of your target body weight. Using the example mentioned earlier, if you want to weigh 175 pounds, you'd need to eat 175 grams of protein each day. Protein is the building block of muscle and the most crucial macronutrient of the three. Many people who start a resistance training program don't get enough protein to properly fuel the repairing and rebuilding process. But beyond giving your body the raw material for packing on lean muscle tissue (and protecting the muscle tissue you already have from being broken down for energy), protein also helps curb your appetite by leaving you feeling fuller, longer.

It also requires the most energy from your body to process. In fact, close to 25 percent of the protein calories you eat is burned off through digestion and absorption. That means that gram for gram, compared to fats and carbohydrates, protein leaves the smallest imprint when it comes to excess calories being stored as unwanted fat.

What type of protein you eat is up to you. The best sources to choose include eggs, fish, lean beef, chicken breast, turkey breast, lean sirloin burger, skim milk, and quality protein powders. Don't feel the need to eat every type—trying to throw back a tuna steak if you're really not a fish lover, for example, is not recommended. Instead, stick with whichever foods you find the most tasty and tolerable.

Fat

Eat 1 gram for every 2 pounds of your target body weight. Using the 175-pound example again, if you want to weigh 175 pounds, you'll need to eat 87.5 grams of fat each day (175 divided by 2).

The biggest misconception many men have is that eating fat makes you fat. In fact, eating "healthy" fats (such as polyunsaturated and monounsaturated) in the right amounts will leave you feeling more satiated, preventing your body from stripping away muscle for energy and making you less likely to binge eat. Fat also plays a major role in other vital functions that are critical for muscle growth, such as helping to minimize excess muscle soreness and improving your recovery time after workouts.

Choose healthy fats that contain omega-3 and omega-6 fatty acids whenever possible. Not only do they both leave you feeling fuller and help you stay strong, but they also come with a list of health benefits, ranging from lowering your risk of heart disease, diabetes, and cancer to boosting your brainpower. Almonds, walnuts, pumpkin seeds, unsalted sunflower seeds, all-natural peanut butter, flaxseed oil, olive oil, any type of fatty fish, and avocados are all great options that contain omega-3 and omega-6 fatty acids and that are easy to add into most meals.

Carbohydrates

Eat whatever's left over in your budget. Simply put, if you want to be a certain weight, as I mentioned in Step 1, you have to eat a certain number of calories. It's easy to hit that magical number by eating carbohydrates, which is why you need to make sure you're eating enough protein and fat first.

Whatever calories are left over, you can spend on carbohydrates. A little math is in order to come up with how many grams of carbohydrates you're allotted each day.

1 Start with the number of grams of protein and fat that you need to eat each day. Each gram of protein equals 4 calories and each gram of fat equals 9 calories. So if your target goal is 175 pounds of lean muscle, those 175 grams of protein will equal 700 calories (175 x 4), while the 87.5 grams of fat will equal 787.5 calories (87.5 x 9).

2 Add up those two numbers: That's how many calories you'll be eating each day from protein and fat alone. (In this case, it's 1,487.5.)

3 Take the total number of calories you need to eat each day (using the 175-pound man example, that would be 2,450 calories) and subtract the number of calories you're eating from protein and fat from that number. In this case, you would subtract 1,487.5 from 2,450 and come up with 962.5.

4 You're almost done! Take that final number and divide it by 4 (which is how many calories are in 1 gram of carbohydrate). That final number is how many grams of carbohydrates you can eat each day. In this case, it's about 241 grams.

Healthy, carbohydrate-rich foods are low in saturated fat, packed with fiber, and loaded with certain essential vitamins and minerals (such as vitamins B_6 and C) that help reduce muscle inflammation and repair and rebuild muscle tissue. But the thing to remember is that not all carbohydrates are created equal.

To maximize your muscle potential, avoid high-glycemic carbohydrates (bread, pasta, white rice, and corn, for example) that elevate your blood sugar and trigger your body to store fat. Instead, opt to eat low-glycemic carbohydrates that take longer to break down and leave you feeling fuller for longer. Try raw, fibrous vegetables (broccoli, spinach, green beans, asparagus, cucumbers, and tomatoes), beans (including black, kidney, pinto, and navy), and grains (such as quinoa, oats, whole wheat bread, and brown rice).

Step #4: Enjoy a Minimeal Before Breakfast

Even though you might have a hard time getting yourself moving when you wake up in the morning, your body is wide awake. And if you're not careful, your body will focus all of its early morning energy on tearing down everything you're desperately trying to build up—your muscles.

You see, by the time you wake up, your body is already in a catabolic state from a lack of food over the previous 6 to 8 hours—a state where your body begins to break down muscle tissue in order to fuel itself. To stop that muscular feast in its tracks, you need to consume some type of protein and carbohydrate snack, especially if you don't plan on having breakfast for at least 30 minutes after waking up. The best solution: Have a small whey protein shake (20 to 30 grams of protein) and ½ cup of fruit. Why whey? It digests quickly, so your body will instantly be able to put it to work.

Need a few good whey protein recipes? Here are some tasty ones. Drink half and save the rest for a snack.

Bananas and Almonds
Blend . . .
6 ounces of fat-free milk
1 tablespoon almond butter
1 scoop chocolate whey protein powder
½ banana
4 ice cubes

The Juicer

Blend . . .

½ cup 1% milk
1 scoop vanilla whey protein powder
¼ cup frozen orange juice concentrate
1 tablespoon plain yogurt
½ banana
3 ice cubes

Strawberry and Banana

Blend . . .

1 scoop vanilla whey protein powder
6 medium strawberries, hulled
1 medium banana
1 cup water
3 ice cubes

Just because you had your wakeup protein shake, that doesn't permit you to skip breakfast. It's a crucial meal for anyone wanting to lose weight and build muscle. The ideal breakfast is high in protein and packed with fiber-rich vegetables and whole grains. That combo will keep you full longer and prevent swings in blood sugar so your energy stays high. Here's a perfect example of a perfect breakfast.

- ▶ Scrambled Eggs and Spinach (Scramble 1 whole egg, 2 egg whites, and ½ cup baby spinach in 1 tablespoon of olive oil.)
- ▶ ¾ cup of oatmeal topped with a handful of chopped walnuts
- ▶ A cup of hot green tea

The eggs provide high-quality, slow-burning protein. Cooking them with heart-healthy olive oil and adding baby spinach, which is high in vitamin A and folate, adds satiating fat and vitamins that improve immune function and cell repair. The oatmeal and walnuts add slow-burning energy and fiber. Washing it down with green tea provides a gentle, sustained caffeine buzz and lowers blood pressure.

Step #5: Take Your Thirst Seriously

For physically active men, drinking the standard, typically recommended eight 8-ounce glasses of water daily won't cut it. A muscle that's dehydrated by as little as 3 percent can experience a 12 percent decrease in strength. Also, exercising while dehydrated has been shown to cause an increase in stress hormones (such as cortisol) and a decrease in the release of testosterone.

The minimum amount of water an avid exerciser should be drinking is 10 to 12 glasses a day (about 96 ounces), but some serious trainers even recommend drinking a minimum of a gallon a day. No matter which amount you decide to consume, you can't afford to assume that your body is fully hydrated because you're counting glasses and gallon containers. Instead, the smartest and easiest rule to follow is to drink all day long and remember a few key things.

CHECK WHEN YOU WAKE UP. Look at the color of your urine first thing in the morning. That's your snapshot of exactly how well hydrated you were the day before. The lighter, the better, and if it's darker than light yellow, you'll know you didn't drink enough the day before.

DRINK AS YOU EXERCISE. How much you perspire can range from 1 pint an hour to as much as three to four times that amount, depending on your intensity, the weather, the temperature, and other factors.

Before you exercise, hydrate yourself with 16 to 24 ounces of water. Then, if possible, sip 4 to 6 ounces every 10 to 15 minutes during your workout, depending on how you feel. But before you take that first sip—and definitely before you start to exercise—weigh yourself. Weighing yourself before and immediately after your workout will help you determine how much water you've lost through sweat. (And if you really mean business, don't step on that scale until you're completely dry and without clothes.) Nearly all of the weight you'll have lost will be water weight, so replace every pound you've lost with about 24 ounces of fluid.

DRINK DURING THE DAY. As I said, if maximum performance is your goal, drinking all day long comes with the territory. You never want to rely on your thirst as a gauge, since by the time you realize you're thirsty, you're most likely already dehydrated or partially dehydrated.

If you need another reason to drink up, consider this: Thirst often disguises itself as hunger because your body draws a large percentage of its water from the foods you eat. Staying hydrated will keep you from eating more than your body needs. And if burning more calories is your mission, whenever possible, make sure that water is on ice. Drinking 16 ounces of chilled water can raise your metabolism by as much as 30 percent—a fat-burning boost that can potentially last up to 90 minutes.

Step #6: Go to Bed with Something in Your Belly

It may seem counterproductive—particularly if your main goal is fat loss—to even consider

FORGET THIS ENTIRE CHAPTER ONCE A WEEK!

If you're sticking with a strict diet, you can blow one meal a week and use that meal as a reward for staying the course. If you do the math, eating 7 meals and snacks each day means eating 49 separate times in 1 week. Throwing out all of these rules and enjoying yourself for one hedonistic meal a week still means that you're following a healthy diet 98 percent of the time, which is more than most people can say, and it won't affect your results in the least.

eating something before going to sleep. Although it's true that eating excessive amounts of calories right before bed will only give your body extra calories it may assume you want to store as body fat, having a small, protein-rich snack immediately before you go to sleep is exactly what you need to preserve your muscle.

As you sleep, your body slips into a catabolic state from not eating for so many hours. The best way to minimize any muscle damage is to consume between 30 and 40 grams of protein at bedtime. Low-fat mozzarella cheese sticks, some cottage cheese, or a protein shake made from casein protein (a type of protein found in dairy products, and the one that takes the longest to digest) will give your stomach something to slowly break down throughout the night, leaving your hard-earned muscles alone.

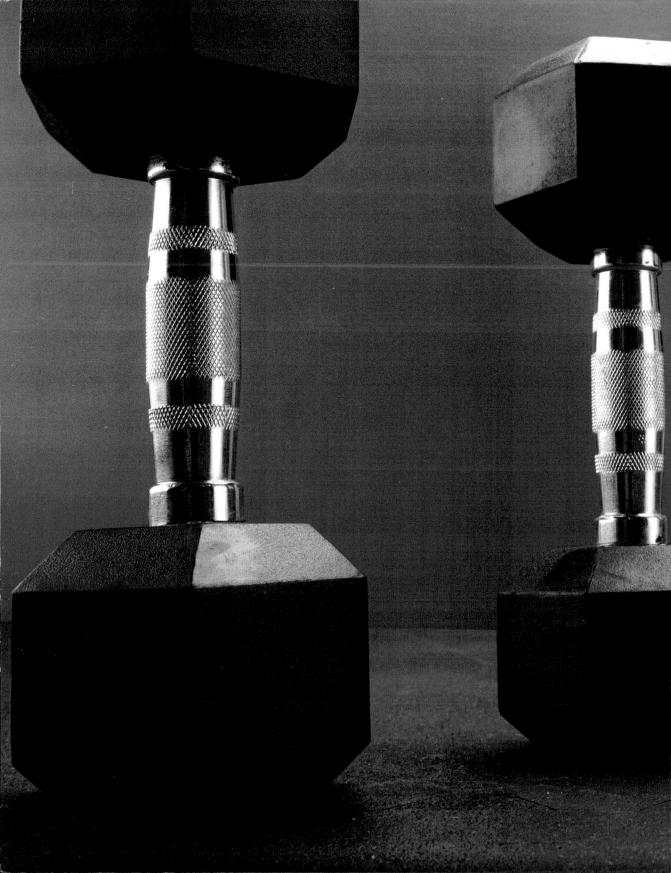

PART TWO
THE
MOVEMENTS

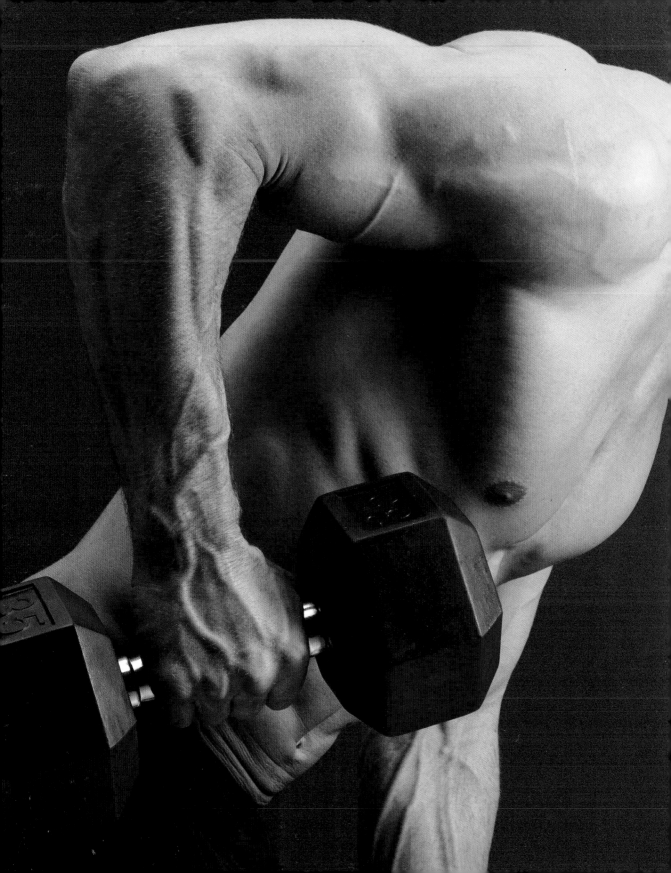

THE BEST DUMBBELL EXERCISES

PUSH, PULL, AND SWING WITH THE MUSCLE-BUILDING KING

If you're like most red-blooded Americans, you already own a pair of these old-school strength tools. Look in your basement or under your bed. If you don't have them, I bet your uncle Jake would be glad to give you his old pair; check in the shed under the "as-seen-on-TV" abs machine he never used.

Dumbbells are simple and simply useful:

A friend of mine takes his out of commission every December to keep his Christmas tree stand from toppling over. But they are especially handy for quick and effective workouts and for taxing every fiber that makes up your musculature. Here's how to rock your range of motion with this classic dynamic duo.

BICEPS CURL

TARGET MUSCLES: biceps

SETUP: Stand tall with your feet hip-width apart and a dumbbell in each hand, palms facing forward. Your arms should be hanging straight at your sides with the dumbbells resting on the fronts of your thighs.

PULL: Keeping your upper arms locked at your sides, slowly pull the dumbbells up until the weights almost reach your shoulders—your palms should now be facing in toward your body. Pause, slowly lower the dumbbells back down, and repeat.

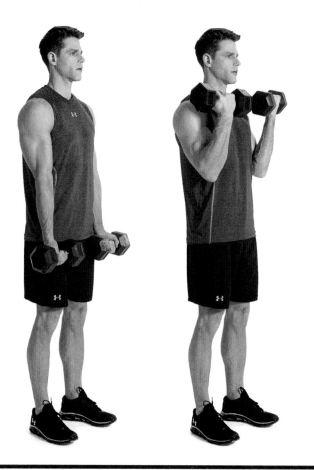

PERFORMANCE POINTERS

STOP BEFORE THE TOP. Don't touch the weights to your shoulders. Doing so may shift your elbows forward. This displaces some of the effort from your biceps to your front deltoids and wrist flexors. Instead, lock your elbows to your sides and stop curling when the weights are a few inches from your shoulders.

CHALLENGE YOUR HANDS. Loop a hand towel around each dumbbell handle and hold the dumbbells as usual. The thicker grip forces your forearms to work harder than they usually do to hold the weight.

DID YOU KNOW?

Good form = better results. Compared with men who performed Curls using only a partial range of motion (that is, they didn't bring the weight all the way down), lifters who used a full range of motion were about 10 percent stronger, according to Brazilian researchers.

OPTIONS

INCLINE HAMMER CURL

Lie on an incline bench set at 45 degrees with your arms hanging straight down to the floor, which angles them behind your body, as opposed to in line with your torso. Your palms should face toward each other. Perform the exercise as explained on the opposite page.

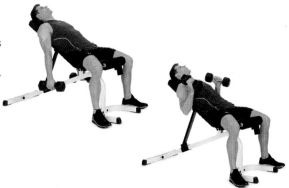

ZOTTMAN CURL

At the top of the curl, rotate your wrists inward until your palms face forward. Lower your arms back down until they're almost locked, then rotate your wrists outward so they once again face forward.

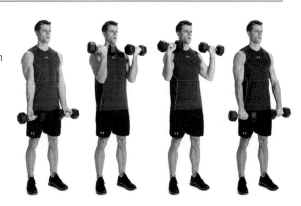

PRONE HAMMER CURL

Grab a dumbbell in each hand and lie with your chest against a bench that's set to a 45-degree incline with your arms hanging straight down to the floor, palms facing in toward each other. This hand positioning places more emphasis on your brachialis, while lying facedown allows the bench to support your upper body, removing momentum from the exercise so that all of the effort is placed on your biceps. Without moving your upper arms, perform a Biceps Curl, keeping a neutral grip. Lower the weights and repeat.

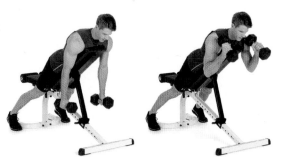

CHEST PRESS

TARGET MUSCLES: chest, shoulders, and triceps

SETUP: Grab a dumbbell in each hand, then lie flat on a bench with your knees bent and your feet flat on the floor. Position the dumbbells along the sides of your chest, elbows pointing toward the floor. Turn the dumbbells so that your palms face toward your feet.

PUSH: Keeping your back flat on the bench, push the dumbbells up until your arms are fully extended above your chest, but don't lock your elbows. (This will keep your chest, shoulders, and triceps in a prolonged state of contraction, which will work them much faster and more thoroughly.) Pause, lower the dumbbells back down to the Setup position, and repeat.

PERFORMANCE POINTERS

DON'T HOLD YOUR BREATH. Inhale as you lower the dumbbells, then exhale as you push them back up into the Setup position.

KEEP YOUR BODY FLAT. Arching your back positions your body to allow other muscles—particularly your triceps—to help lift the weight, which reduces effort from your chest while placing your lower back at risk of strain. Keep it on the bench.

ADD A FLEX AT THE TOP. Once you've pushed the weights up, squeeze your pectorals together as if you were trying to squeeze a quarter between them.

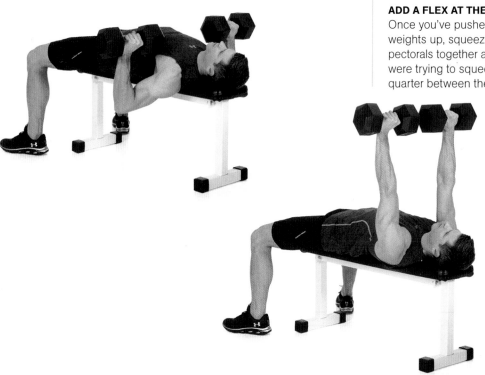

OPTIONS

FLOOR PRESS

Lie flat on the floor, holding the weights with straight arms above your shoulders. As you lower the weights, stop when your upper arms gently touch the floor, then press back up.

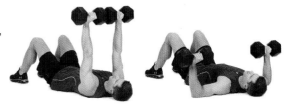

INCLINE CHEST PRESS

Choose a pair of dumbbells that are 10 to 20 percent lighter than you would to do the Chest Press. Lie on an incline bench set at between 30 and 45 degrees. The angle of the bench changes the ratio of effort, sharing more of the stress with your shoulders, which means you'll lift less weight. Perform the exercise as explained on the opposite page.

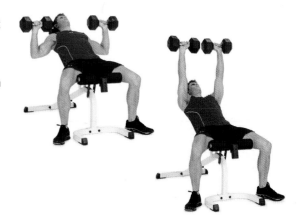

ALTERNATING CHEST PRESS

Slowly raise one dumbbell until your arm is fully extended but not locked. Pause, and as you lower the weight back to the starting position, raise the dumbbell in your other hand. Continue to alternate.

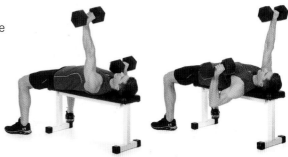

CHEST FLY

TARGET MUSCLES: chest and front deltoids

SETUP: Grab a dumbbell in each hand, then lie flat on a bench with your knees bent and your feet flat on the floor. Raise your arms straight up above your chest with your elbows slightly bent and your palms facing toward your feet.

PULL: Keeping your arms in this position, sweep the dumbbells down and out to your sides in an arc until the dumbbells are at about chest level. Pause, pull your arms back up to the Setup position, and repeat.

PERFORMANCE POINTER

KEEP ELBOWS LOCKED.
If you bend your elbows more as you bring them down, you turn the exercise into a pushing movement (essentially a Bench Press) instead of a pulling movement, making it less difficult. To keep that from happening, bend your arms slightly *before* you perform the move, then keep your elbows locked in that bent position throughout the exercise.

OPTION

INCLINE CHEST FLY
Lie on an incline bench set at between 30 and 45 degrees. Perform the exercise as explained at left.

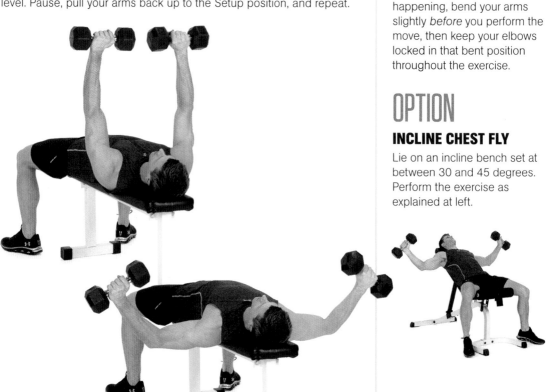

CRUNCH

TARGET MUSCLE: rectus abdominis

SETUP: Lie flat on your back on a mat or carpeted surface, knees bent and feet flat on the floor. Use both hands to grab a dumbbell by its ends, and rest it on your chest.

PULL: Keeping the dumbbell in place, slowly pull your head and shoulders 4 to 6 inches off the floor and toward your knees. Pause as you contract your core muscles, lower yourself back down, and repeat.

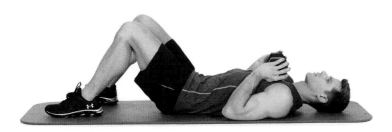

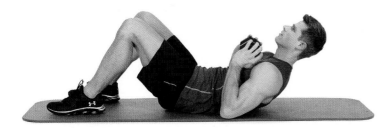

PERFORMANCE POINTERS

DON'T PEEL OFF THE FLOOR. Instead of rolling up, concentrate on folding your upper body forward, keeping your shoulders and upper back straight (not rounded) as you crunch.

NEVER HOOK YOUR FEET. Whenever you anchor your feet during abdominal exercises, you take stress away from your abs and transfer more of the effort onto your hip flexors, the muscles that attach the front of your torso to your legs.

OPTION

LONG-ARM CRUNCH
Extend your arms so the dumbbell is above your chest. Perform the exercise as explained at left.

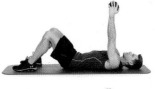

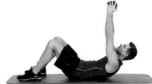

CLEAN AND PRESS

TARGET MUSCLES: back, chest, core, glutes, legs, shoulders, and triceps

SETUP: Stand tall with your feet hip-width apart and a dumbbell in each hand, palms facing in. Your arms should be hanging in front of you with the dumbbells resting on the fronts of your thighs.

PUSH, PULL (AND SWING): Push your hips back and bend your knees slightly so the dumbbells drop to just above your knees. In one move, explosively swing the dumbbells upward toward your shoulders, push your hips forward, and drive your feet into the floor to straighten your legs. As the dumbbells come above waist height, bend your knees to help "catch" them in front of your shoulders. Quickly push your heels into the floor as you simultaneously push the dumbbells over your head. Reverse the motion to lower the dumbbells into the Setup position, and repeat.

PERFORMANCE POINTER

KEEP YOUR FEET FLAT.
You should be able to wiggle your toes. That will tell you that your weight is loaded more along the back of your body.

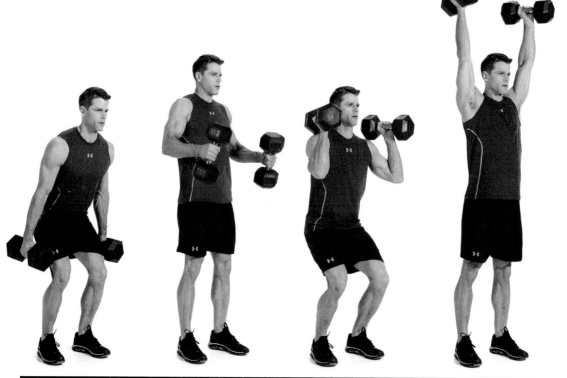

FRONT SQUAT

TARGET MUSCLES: legs (primarily the quadriceps)

SETUP: Stand tall with your feet hip-width apart and a dumbbell in each hand. Raise both dumbbells up to your chest, palms facing in, and place one end of each dumbbell on the front of each shoulder. Your elbows will be pointing down.

PUSH: Keeping your torso straight, slowly push your hips back, bend your knees, and squat down until your thighs are parallel to the floor or lower. Push yourself back up until your legs are straight but not locked, and repeat.

DON'T SUFFER IN SILENCE. If resting the dumbbells on your shoulders is uncomfortable, try wrapping a towel across the front of your chest and draping the ends over your shoulders to cushion the weight.

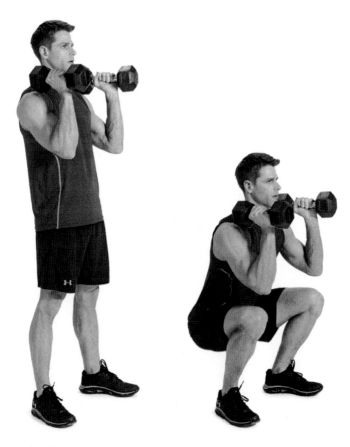

SQUAT

TARGET MUSCLES: glutes, hamstrings, quadriceps, and calves

SETUP: Stand tall with your feet shoulder-width apart and a dumbbell in each hand, palms facing in. Your arms should hang down at your sides and your knees should not be locked.

PUSH: Keeping your head and back straight, push your hips back and slowly squat down until your thighs are parallel to the floor. (Your knees should be directly above your toes; avoid letting them extend past your feet.) Push yourself back up into the Setup position, and repeat.

PERFORMANCE POINTERS

LOOK STRAIGHT AHEAD.
Don't stare down as you squat. Looking down during the exercise (or moving your head to look left or right) will affect your balance, which can make the exercise more difficult to do.

STRAIGHTEN YOUR LEGS. DON'T LOCK YOUR KNEES.
Locking them takes the load off of your muscles and redirects the stress to your knee joints.

PUSH THE FLOOR AWAY.
This tactic will allow you to better engage the muscles in your legs.

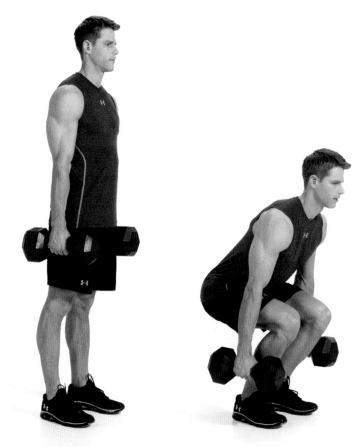

OPTIONS

JUMP SQUAT

Perform the exercise as described on the opposite page, but after you lower yourself into a squat, jump as high as you can. Land softly, with your knees bent. Return to the Setup position, and repeat.

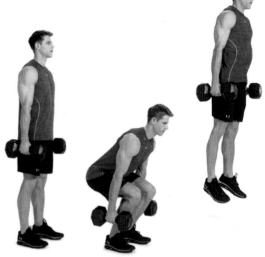

BULGARIAN ISOMETRIC SQUAT

Stand about 3 feet away from a weight bench, with your back to it. Grab a dumbbell in each hand, arms hanging at your sides. Extend your right leg back and rest your right foot on top of the bench—the top of your foot should be flat on the top of the bench. Bend your left knee and lower yourself down until your left thigh is parallel to the floor. Pause, straighten your left leg, and repeat. Perform the required number of repetitions, switch sides, and repeat.

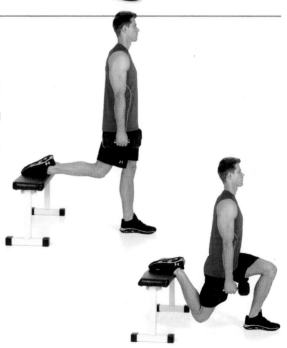

DEADLIFT

TARGET MUSCLES: glutes, legs, lower back, trapezius, abs, and calves

SETUP: Stand tall with your feet hip-width apart and a pair of heavy dumbbells on the floor in front of you. Bend your knees and grab the dumbbells with palms facing your body.

PULL: With your chest held up and away from your body and your back flat, slowly pull the dumbbells off the floor by standing up as you thrust your hips forward. Pause, lower the dumbbells back down to the floor, and repeat.

PERFORMANCE POINTERS

STRAIGHTEN YOUR LEGS. Before you start to pull the weight from the floor, extend your legs. Feeling tension from the dumbbells before you lift them distributes the effort of the exercise evenly throughout your muscles.

KEEP YOUR ARMS STRAIGHT. Resist the urge to raise your shoulders or bend your elbows as you go. The dumbbells should stay close to your body as you lift until your legs are straight but not locked.

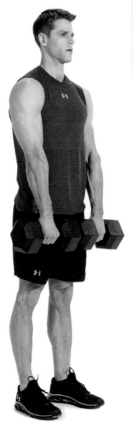
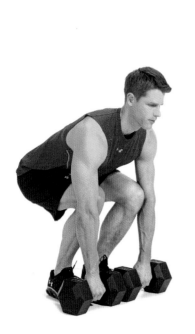

OPTIONS

NEUTRAL-GRIP DEADLIFT

Grab the dumbbells with a neutral grip—palms facing in toward each other. Perform the exercise as explained on the opposite page.

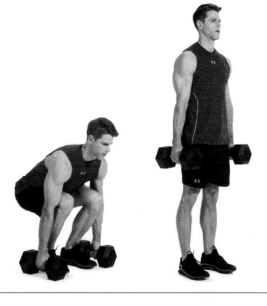

SUMO DEADLIFT

Place a heavy dumbbell on its end and stand in front of it with your feet wider than shoulder-width apart and your toes pointed out to the sides. Bend your knees, reach down, and grab the dumbbell with both hands, wrapping your fingers over the sides of the bell, palms facing down. Perform the exercise as explained on the opposite page.

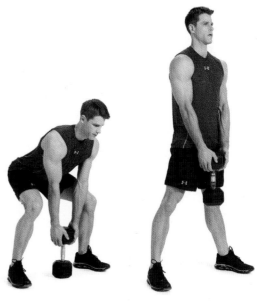

ROMANIAN DEADLIFT

TARGET MUSCLES: back, glutes, and hamstrings

SETUP: Stand tall with your feet shoulder-width apart, knees slightly bent, holding a pair of dumbbells, palms facing your body. Your arms should be hanging down in front of your legs.

PULL: Slowly push your hips back and sit back, allowing your knees to bend more as you bend forward (keeping your chest up) and lower the dumbbells to just below your knees. Pull your torso back into the Setup position, then repeat.

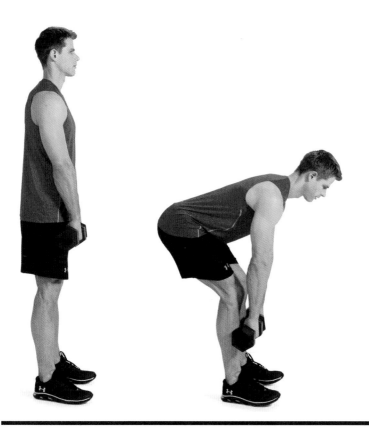

PERFORMANCE POINTER

STAY TIGHT.
Keep the weights as close to your body as possible. This will focus all of the effort onto your hamstrings, not your lower back.

OPTION

SINGLE-LEG ROMANIAN DEADLIFT

Lift one foot an inch or two off the floor behind you so that you're balancing on the other foot. Holding this position, slowly shift your hips backward and bend forward until your back and back leg are almost parallel to the floor. Allow your arms to hang straight down. Raise your torso back up into a standing position and perform the required number of repetitions. Switch legs and repeat the exercise.

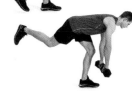

STRAIGHT-LEG DEADLIFT

TARGET MUSCLES: back, glutes, hamstrings, and core

SETUP: Stand tall with your feet hip-width apart, a slight bend in the knees, and a dumbbell in each hand, palms facing backward. Your arms should be hanging straight down in front of your thighs.

PULL: Keeping your back flat, legs straight, and knees unlocked, bend forward from your waist and lower your torso until it's almost parallel to the floor. Reverse the motion to return to the Setup position, and repeat.

PERFORMANCE POINTER

DON'T ROUND YOUR BACK. Your low back should stay naturally arched during the movement.

OPTION

SINGLE-LEG STRAIGHT-LEG DEADLIFT

Balance yourself on one foot by lifting your other foot a few inches off the floor behind you. Without changing the bend in your back leg, bend at your waist and lower your torso until it's almost parallel to the floor while raising your back leg. Perform the pull portion as explained.

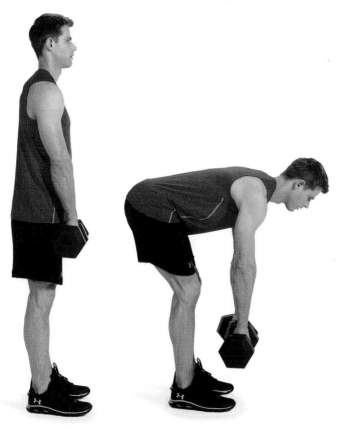

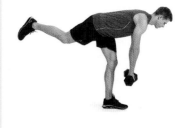

LATERAL RAISE

TARGET MUSCLES: medial deltoids
(the sides of your shoulders)

SETUP: Stand tall with your feet shoulder-width apart and a dumbbell in each hand, palms facing forward. Your arms should be hanging at your sides with a slight bend in your elbows.

PULL: Keeping your elbows slightly bent, slowly pull your arms up and out from your sides until they are parallel to the floor—your body should resemble the letter T. Pause, slowly lower your arms back down to your sides, and repeat.

PERFORMANCE POINTERS

STOP AT PARALLEL.
Raise your arms slowly to avoid allowing momentum to raise them higher than parallel, which can cause injury.

DON'T ROTATE YOUR ARMS.
Some people think turning your shoulders forward makes the move more effective, but it only increases your risk of injuring them.

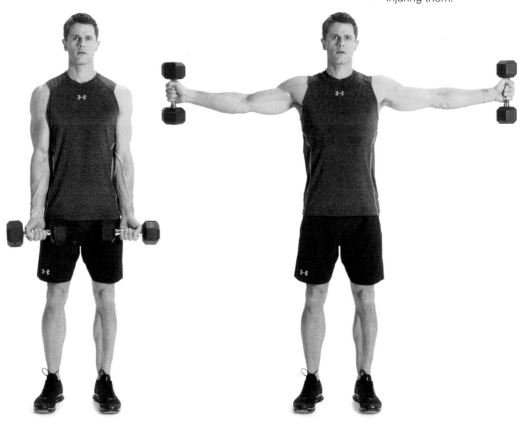

OPTIONS

SEATED (OR KNEELING) LATERAL RAISE

Choose a weight that's 40 to 50 percent lighter than you might use for a Lateral Raise and sit on a weight bench (or kneel on a mat or carpeted floor) with your arms hanging straight down at your sides, palms facing forward. Perform the exercise as described on the opposite page.

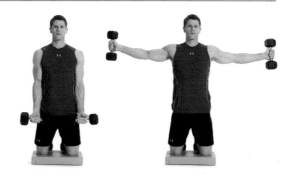

LATERAL T-RAISE

Bend your arms at 90 degrees. Hold this arm position as you perform the exercise as described on the opposite page.

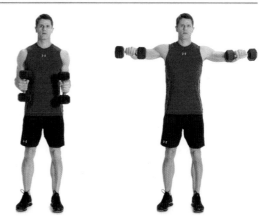

SINGLE-ARM LATERAL RAISE

Instead of raising both arms simultaneously, raise one arm at a time. This trick will force your core muscles to work harder in order to keep you balanced as you go.

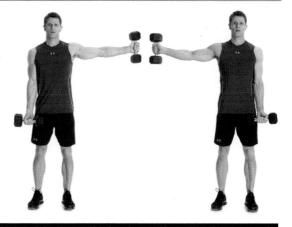

REAR LATERAL RAISE

TARGET MUSCLES: rear deltoids, rotator cuff muscles, and upper and middle back

SETUP: Stand tall with your feet hip- to shoulder-width apart and a light dumbbell in each hand. Bend at your waist and lean forward until your back is flat and as parallel to the floor as possible. Let your arms hang down directly below you, palms facing in.

PULL: Keeping your back fixed in this position and your arms straight and elbows unlocked, slowly pull the weights out to your sides until your arms are parallel to the floor. Pause, then slowly lower your arms back down into the Setup position.

PERFORMANCE POINTER

DON'T LIFT YOUR TORSO. If you rise as you lift, you're using momentum and your lower back to cheat the weights upward. Instead, focus on making sure that only your arms are moving during the exercise.

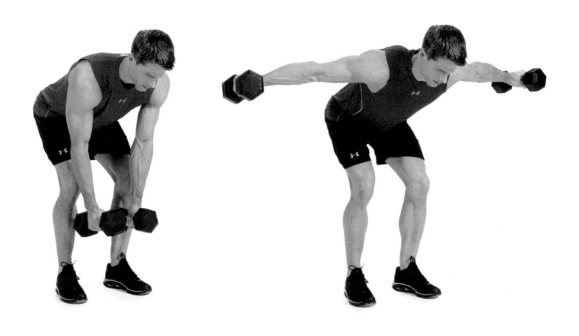

SINGLE-LEG STANDING CALF RAISE

TARGET MUSCLES: calves

SETUP: Hold a dumbbell in your right hand and stand on a stable surface that's 6 to 12 inches tall (such as a step or a block of wood). Place your foot on the step so that just the ball of your foot is on the edge and your heel is hanging off.

Grab the edge of a wall with your left hand for balance if necessary, then tuck your left foot behind your right ankle so your weight is resting on the ball of your right foot.

PUSH: Slowly push through the ball of your right foot and raise your right heel up as high as possible. Pause, slowly lower your right heel down as far as you can, and repeat. Perform the required number of repetitions, switch sides, and repeat.

PERFORMANCE POINTER

TRY IT SEATED.
Your calves are made up of two different muscles—the gastrocnemius and the soleus. Performing the exercise with a straight leg (as shown) primarily works the gastrocnemius, but bending your knee places more stress on your soleus. Try a set of Seated Calf Raises with your foot on a weight plate and a dumbbell on the knee of the working leg.

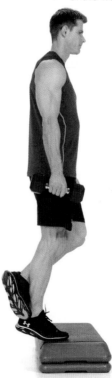

LUNGE

TARGET MUSCLES: quadriceps, hamstrings, glutes, and calves

SETUP: Stand tall with your feet hip-width apart and a dumbbell in each hand, palms facing in. Your arms should be hanging at your sides.

PUSH: Take a big step forward with your left foot and lower your body until your left thigh is parallel to the floor. Your right knee should be an inch or two off the floor and should be bent at a 90-degree angle, and only the ball of your right foot should be on the floor.

Quickly reverse the motion by pushing yourself back into the Setup position, then step forward with your right foot, lowering your body until your left knee is bent at 90 degrees. Step back into the Setup position and repeat.

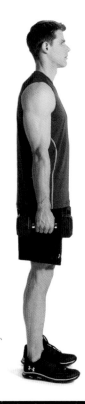
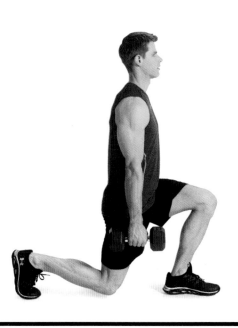

LISTEN TO YOUR KNEES.
If stepping forward bothers them, try performing a Reverse Lunge by taking a big step backward, instead. Lower yourself down by bending the knee of your forward leg and sinking down until your forward thigh is parallel to the floor.

LOOK FORWARD.
Don't look down at your feet. Staring at the floor can cause you to lose your balance.

NARROW YOUR STANCE.
The closer your feet are to each other, the harder your core muscles will have to work to stabilize your body.

WATCH YOUR KNEES.
Never let your knee travel past your toes as you lunge. Your forward knee should end up directly over your foot, so that your leg forms a 90-degree angle.

OPTIONS

T-PUSHUP

Perform the exercise as explained on the opposite page, but as you push yourself up, rotate your body to the right, lift the dumbbell in your right hand off the floor, and extend it straight up toward the ceiling. (Your body will look like a T.) Twist back down, place the dumbbell back on the floor, then do another Pushup. As you push yourself up, rotate to the left and extend the dumbbell in your left hand up to the ceiling. Keep alternating from right to left.
Extra credit: Includes a Swing!

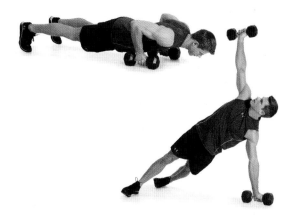

PUSHUP DRAG

Start in a Pushup position with a dumbbell on the floor next to your left side. Bend your elbows, lower your chest toward the floor, and then push yourself back up until your arms are straight. Shift your weight to your left arm as you reach your right arm underneath your body to grab the dumbbell. Drag the dumbbell underneath you until it rests at your right side. Get back into a pushup position and repeat, this time dragging the weight to your left side with your left hand as you shift your weight onto your right arm.
Extra credit: Includes a Swing!

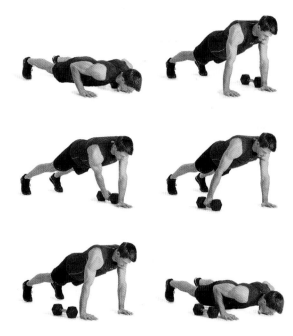

PUSH PRESS

TARGET MUSCLES: shoulders, legs, triceps, upper trapezius, and core

SETUP: Stand tall with your feet shoulder-width apart and a heavy dumbbell in each hand. Hold the weights up in front of your shoulders with palms facing each other.

PUSH: Keeping your back straight and eyes forward, squat down about 6 inches, then explosively push up with your legs as you push the dumbbells straight above your shoulders. Pause, slowly lower the dumbbells back down to the Setup position, and repeat.

PERFORMANCE POINTER

PUSH THROUGH YOUR HEELS. This will give you more power when pushing the weights directly overhead.

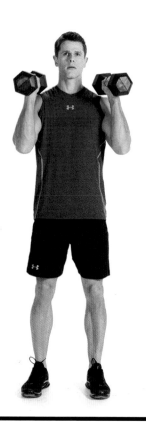
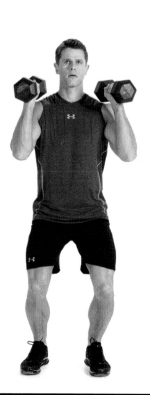
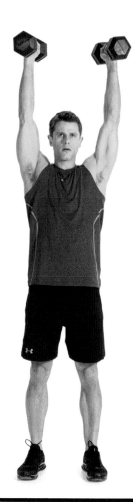

SHRUG

TARGET MUSCLES: upper trapezius

SETUP: Stand tall with your feet hip- to shoulder-width apart and a heavy dumbbell in each hand, palms facing in. Your arms should be hanging down at your sides.

PULL: Without moving your arms, raise your shoulders up toward your ears as high as you can. Lower them back down, then repeat.

PERFORMANCE POINTERS

KEEP YOUR ARMS STRAIGHT.
Bending your arms as you raise the weights would shift effort to other muscles that will tire out before your upper trapezius muscles do.

DON'T ROLL YOUR SHOULDERS.
Your upper trapezius muscles are designed to pull your shoulders up and down—not backward or forward—so doing so could cause neck strain.

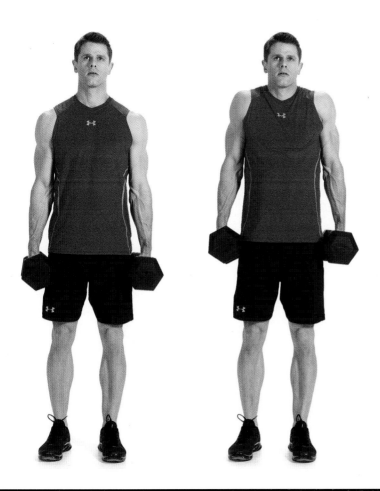

DID YOU KNOW?

You can increase your metabolism by at least 8.5 percent if you eat 18 grams of protein prior to a training session, according to research in the journal *Medicine and Science in Sports and Exercise.*

REVERSE CRUNCH

TARGET MUSCLE: rectus abdominis

SETUP: Lie flat on your back on a mat or carpeted surface with your knees bent and feet together and flat on the floor. Place a light dumbbell between your thighs close to your knees and squeeze it so it stays in place throughout the exercise. Stretch your arms out to your sides, palms down, for support.

PULL: Holding the dumbbell tightly in place and keeping your feet together, slowly pull your knees up to your chest so that your hips and lower back lift off the floor. Pause, lower your legs back down, and repeat.

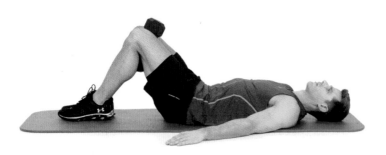

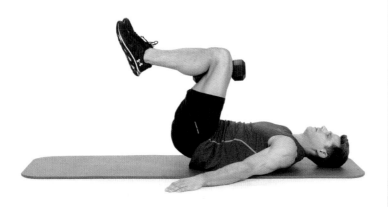

PERFORMANCE POINTERS

CONTRACT YOUR CORE.
Contracting your abdominal muscles before you start and keeping them that way throughout the exercise will help support your lower back.

GO SLOWLY.
The slower you perform this exercise, the longer your abdominal muscles will remain under tension. Imagine that you're trying to empty—as slowly as possible—a bucket of water that's attached to your pelvis.

OPTION

DOUBLE CRUNCH
Use both hands to hold another light dumbbell by its ends, and rest it on your chest with your elbows flared out to your sides. Holding both dumbbells in place, slowly pull your head and shoulders off the floor as you simultaneously pull your knees up to your chest. Pause, lower, and repeat.

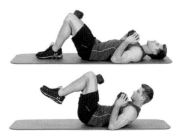

KNEELING TWIST

TARGET MUSCLES: core

SETUP: Kneel on a mat or carpeted surface. Holding a light dumbbell with both hands, lean back until your torso is at a 45-degree angle. Extend your arms straight out in front of you, parallel to the floor.

SWING: Keeping your core muscles tight and arms straight, rotate your torso to the right as far as you can, then rotate to the left as far as you can. Return to the Setup position (that's 1 rep) and repeat.

PERFORMANCE POINTER

BRACE YOUR CORE.
Avoid injury by tightening your abs and twisting slowly.

OPTION

RUSSIAN TWIST

Instead of kneeling, sit on the floor with your knees bent and heels on the floor. Without moving your legs, perform the exercise from side to side as described. As another option, raise your feet an inch or two off the floor and keep them there while you perform the exercise as explained.

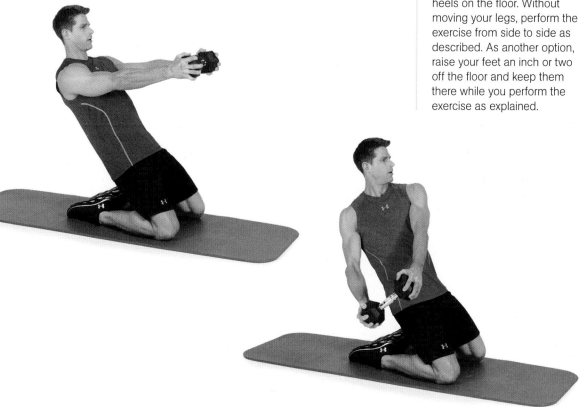

SIDE PLANK

TARGET MUSCLES: core

SETUP: Lie on your left side on a mat or carpeted surface with your legs straight and prop your upper body up on your left elbow and forearm so your elbow is positioned directly underneath your shoulder. Grab a light dumbbell with your right hand and extend your right arm toward the ceiling, perpendicular to the floor.

PUSH: Keeping your right arm extended, tighten your core muscles and push up your hips until your body forms a straight line from your ankles to your shoulders, keeping your head in line with your body. Hold this position for the required amount of time, then switch sides and repeat.

KEEP YOUR CORE TIGHT. Brace your core by contracting your abs forcefully, then hold them in that contracted state. (Imagine you're expecting to be punched in the stomach at any time.)

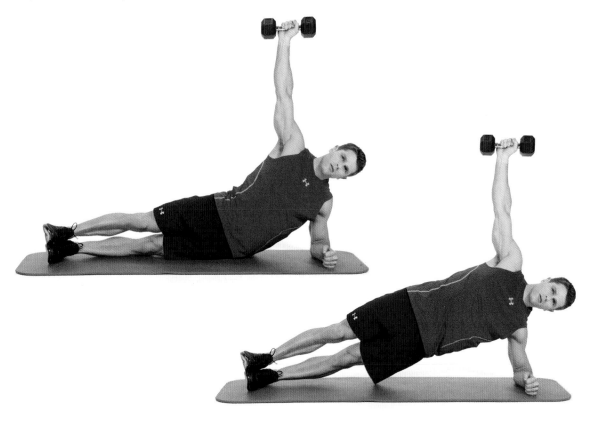

STANDING TWIST

TARGET MUSCLES: core

SETUP: Stand tall with your feet shoulder-width apart and use both hands to hold a dumbbell by its ends. Bend your arms so that they're roughly at 90-degree angles, hold the dumbbell in front of your chest, and tuck your upper arms into your sides.

SWING: Keeping your upper arms locked in place, twist at your waist and swing your torso as far left as you can. As you go, raise your right heel off the floor and pivot off the ball of your right foot. Reverse the motion by twisting at your waist and swinging your torso as far right as you can, raising your left heel and pivoting off the ball of your left foot. Return to the Setup position and repeat.

PERFORMANCE POINTER

DON'T TWIST TOO FAST.
If you do, you'll place your lower back at risk of injury. Instead, perform the motion at a normal pace.

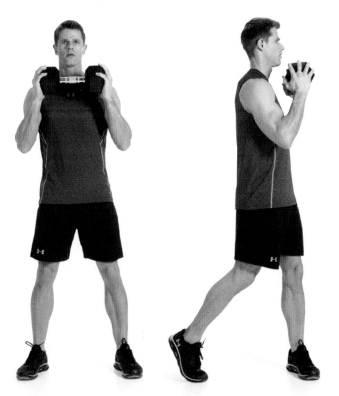

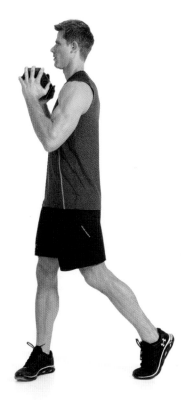

STEPUP

TARGET MUSCLES: glutes, hamstrings, quadriceps, and calves

SETUP: Stand in front of an exercise bench or step with your feet shoulder-width apart and a dumbbell in each hand, palms facing in. Your arms should be hanging at your sides.

PUSH: Keeping your back straight, place your left foot firmly on the bench and push yourself up (using only your left leg) until your right foot is able to step up on top of the bench—but don't place your right foot on the bench. Pause, then take 2 seconds to lower your right foot back down to the ground so that it lands softly.

Perform all the required repetitions with your left foot on the bench, then repeat with your right foot on the bench.

PERFORMANCE POINTER

BRUSH THE FLOOR.
If you find that you are cheating by pushing off with your back foot, try to just brush the floor with your toes instead of placing your foot completely on the floor.

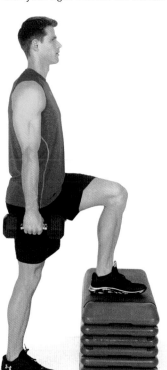
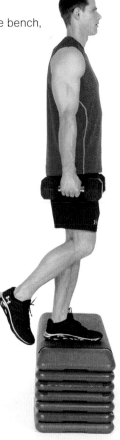

OPTION

CROSSOVER STEPUP

Hold a dumbbell in each hand and stand next to a bench or step that's about knee-height. If your left leg is next to the step (as shown), raise your right foot and cross it in front of your left leg. Place it flat on the step. Push off with your left leg and straighten your right leg until you are standing on your right leg on top of the step. Step onto the floor with your left foot and then your right foot. Reverse the movement by crossing your left foot in front of your right leg and placing that foot on the step. Completing the move equals 1 repetition. Continue for the required reps.

TWO-ARM ROW

TARGET MUSCLES: latissimus dorsi, lower back, middle trapezius, and rhomboids

SETUP: Stand tall with your feet hip-width apart, knees slightly bent, and a dumbbell in each hand, palms facing in. Keeping your back flat, bend forward at your waist until your torso is almost parallel to the floor—your arms should extend straight down below you.

PULL: Without moving your upper body, pull the dumbbells up to the sides of your torso and squeeze your shoulder blades together. Pause, lower the dumbbells back down, and repeat.

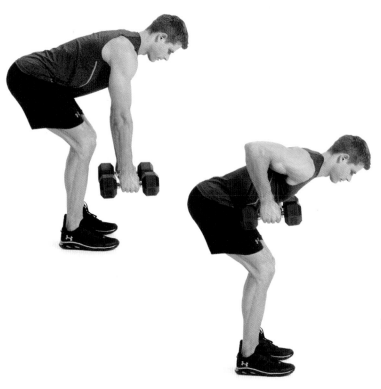

PERFORMANCE POINTERS

LOOK AT THE FLOOR.
Keep your head, neck, and spine in line with each other.

PULL SHOULDERS BACK.
Keep them that way throughout the exercise. This activates your middle- and upper-back muscles.

HAVE A BALL.
Imagine you have one between your shoulder blades. Try to squeeze that ball with your shoulder blades as you pull the weights up.

OPTION

SINGLE-LEG ROW

Stand with a light dumbbell in each hand. Bend your right knee to lift your right foot behind you, then slowly bend forward at your waist until your back is almost parallel to the floor, and then row.

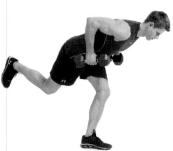

BENT-OVER ROW

TARGET MUSCLES: biceps, latissimus dorsi, lower back, posterior deltoids, and trapezius

SETUP: Stand tall with your left side to an exercise bench and a dumbbell in your right hand. Rest your left hand and knee on the bench, bend at your waist, and let your right arm hang down toward the floor, palm facing in toward the bench.

PULL: Draw the weight up close to your body until it reaches the side of your torso. Pause, lower the dumbbell back down until your arm is straight, and repeat. Perform the required number of repetitions, switch sides, and repeat.

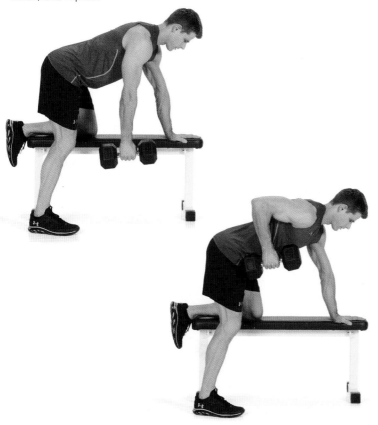

PERFORMANCE POINTER

DON'T TWIST YOUR TORSO. If you do while lifting the dumbbell, your lower back and core muscles will take on some of the effort, preventing you from working your upper back efficiently.

OPTION

LAWNMOWER PULL

Hold a dumbbell in your right hand and stand in a split stance, left foot in front of your right by about 2 feet, left arm hanging at your side. Bend your left knee and your hips until your torso is at about a 45-degree angle, letting the dumbbell hang at arm's length. In one move, explosively straighten your left leg and thrust your hips forward as you rotate your torso, pivot your feet, and pull the weight to your shoulder. Reverse the move and repeat. After you've performed the required number of repetitions, switch sides and repeat.

WOODCHOP

TARGET MUSCLES: abdominals, lower back, and shoulders

SETUP: Stand tall with your feet shoulder-width apart and a light dumbbell in both hands with a hand-over-hand grip. Both of your arms should be extended above your right shoulder.

SWING: Keeping your knees slightly bent, quickly twist your torso to your left and bend at your waist as you draw your arms across and down—the dumbbell should end up just outside of your left knee or ankle. (You should move as if you're chopping wood.) Quickly reverse the movement with the same intensity, and repeat. Perform the required number of repetitions, switch sides, and repeat.

PERFORMANCE POINTER

STICK WITH PERFECT FORM. Your arms should stay nearly straight, and your core muscles should remain tight throughout the exercise.

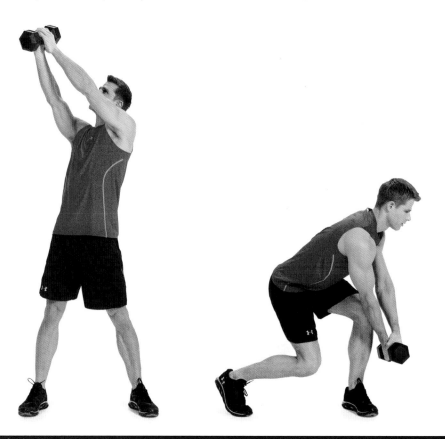

OPTIONS

SINGLE-LEG WOODCHOP

Hold a light dumbbell with a hand-over-hand grip and your arms extended above your right shoulder. Bend your left knee 90 degrees to lift your left foot behind you. Balancing on your right leg, perform the exercise as explained on the opposite page. Do the required number of repetitions, switch sides, and repeat.

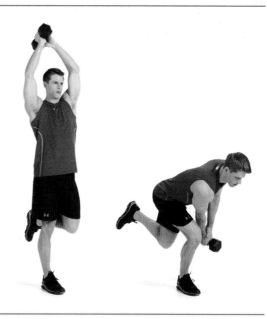

REVERSE WOODCHOP

Bend your knees and lean forward, positioning the dumbbell along the outside of your left calf. Straighten your legs and use your core to swing the weight up and over your right shoulder, then bring the weight back down. Perform the required number of repetitions, switch sides, and repeat.

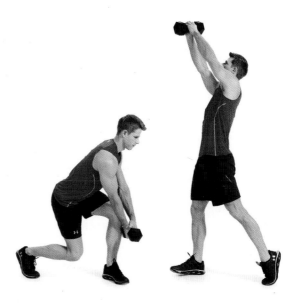

LYING TRICEPS EXTENSION

TARGET MUSCLES: triceps

SETUP: Grab a light dumbbell in each hand, then lie flat on an exercise bench with your knees bent and feet flat on the floor. Straighten your arms above you so that the weights are above your head, palms facing in.

PUSH: Without moving your upper arms, bend your elbows and slowly lower the dumbbells until they reach the sides of your head. Slowly push the weights above you, and repeat.

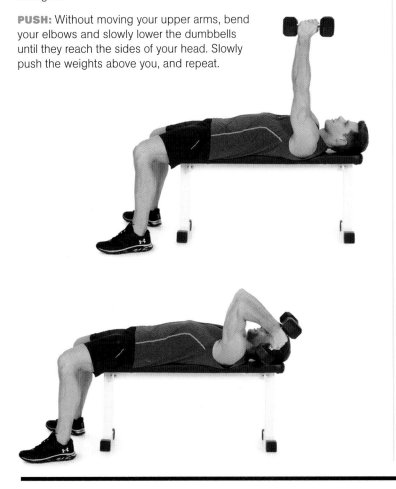

PERFORMANCE POINTER

DON'T MOVE UPPER ARMS. Before you begin, point your arms up at the ceiling, and then concentrate on keeping your upper arms in place.

OPTION

TATE PRESS

Lie flat on an exercise bench holding a dumbbell in each hand. Extend your arms above your chest, palms facing toward your feet with the ends of the weights touching each other. Bend your elbows so they extend out to the sides and lower one end of each dumbbell to the center of your chest. Push the weights back up without letting the dumbbells come apart, and repeat.

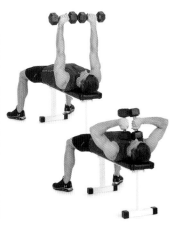

SINGLE-ARM TRICEPS KICKBACK

TARGET MUSCLES: triceps

SETUP: Stand tall with your left side to an exercise bench and a dumbbell in your right hand. Rest your left hand and knee on the bench, bend at your waist, and let your right arm hang down toward the floor, palm facing in toward the bench. Pull your right elbow up so that your upper arm is in line with your back. Your arm should be at a 90-degree angle, knuckles pointing toward the floor, palm facing in.

PUSH: Without moving your upper arm, slowly extend your arm straight back. Pause, reverse the movement, and return to the Setup position. Perform the required number of repetitions, switch sides, and repeat.

PERFORMANCE POINTERS

GO SLOWLY.
Avoid moving your upper arm. Slowly straighten your forearm and do not bend your wrist.

STARE STRAIGHT DOWN.
Don't turn your head to the side to see if your arm is straight, because this can sometimes cause neck stress. Instead, look to make sure your upper arm is parallel to the floor before you begin the exercise, then keep your eyes on the bench for the rest of the movement.

OPTION

TWO-ARM TRICEPS KICKBACK

Stand straight with your knees unlocked, your feet shoulder-width apart, and a light dumbbell in each hand. Keeping your back flat, bend forward at your waist until your torso is parallel to the floor, then raise and lower both dumbbells at the same time.

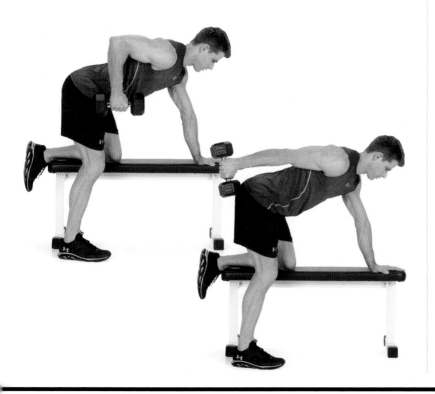

OVERHEAD TRICEPS EXTENSION

TARGET MUSCLES: triceps

SETUP: Stand straight, feet shoulder-width apart, holding a dumbbell in both hands. Push the dumbbell over your head and hold it so that either both hands wrap around its middle or your palms are flat against the inside plate.

PUSH: Without moving your upper arms, slowly bend your elbows and lower the dumbbell behind your head as far as possible. Push the dumbbell back overhead until your arms are straight, and repeat.

KEEP YOUR CORE TIGHT. Don't allow your torso to lean backward or forward. Bracing your core as if you expect someone to punch you will help keep your body straight.

FOCUS ON YOUR FOREARMS. Slowly lower the weights to ensure proper form. Your forearms should lower to at least parallel to the floor.

RESIST MOVEMENT. Keep your upper arms stationary. Your elbows shouldn't change position throughout the move.

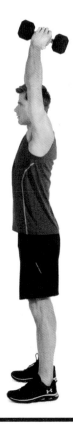
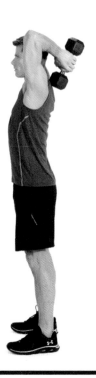

PULLOVER

TARGET MUSCLES: latissimus dorsi and middle trapezius

SETUP: Grab a dumbbell and lie on a flat bench with your feet flat on the floor. Shift yourself so that the top of your head is even with the very end of the bench. Wrap your hands around the inside end of the dumbbell, then press it above your chest.

PULL: Slowly move the dumbbell in an arc over your head, lowering it until your upper arms are in line with your head. Pause, pull the dumbbell back into the Setup position above your chest, and repeat.

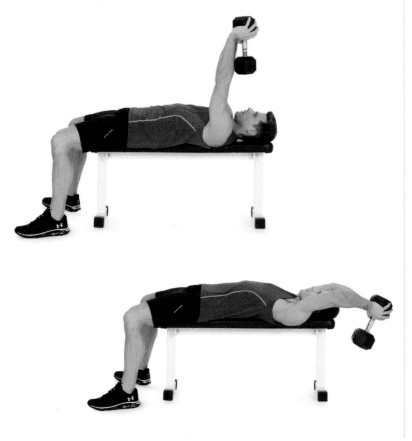

PERFORMANCE POINTER

NEVER BEND YOUR ARMS. If you do, you're cheating the weights upward by using your triceps muscles.

OPTION

CROSS-BENCH PULLOVER

Position yourself perpendicular to a weight bench and lie back so that only your shoulders and upper back are resting on it—your head will hang off one side while your body will be on the opposite side, knees bent at 90 degrees and feet flat on the floor. Your body should be straight from your knees to your head. Perform the exercise as explained.

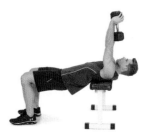

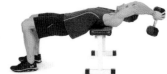

STANDING SHOULDER PRESS

TARGET MUSCLES: shoulders, triceps, and upper trapezius

SETUP: Stand tall with your feet shoulder-width apart and a dumbbell in each hand, just outside your shoulders, palms facing in.

PUSH: Keeping your back straight and eyes forward, push the weights up over your head until your arms are straight, elbows locked. Lower the weights to the Setup position and repeat.

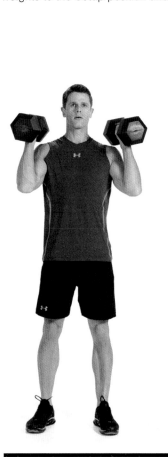
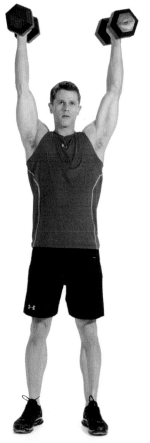

PERFORMANCE POINTERS

WORK FROM TOP DOWN.
The weights should travel in a straight line, starting from your shoulders. Don't push them up at an inward angle that allows them to touch at the top of the movement.

SQUEEZE YOUR GLUTES.
By doing so, your body is forced into a position that automatically stabilizes your spine.

OPTION

SINGLE-ARM SHOULDER PRESS

Stand tall, holding one dumbbell just outside your shoulder with your arm bent and your palm facing your shoulder. Perform the required number of repetitions as explained, switch sides, and repeat.

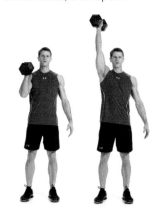

HANG PULL

TARGET MUSCLES: biceps, calves, core, glutes, hamstrings, posterior deltoids, quadriceps, and upper and lower back

SETUP: Stand with your feet shoulder-width apart and holding a dumbbell in each hand against your thighs using an overhand grip (palms facing in). Push your hips back, bend forward slightly, and bend your knees slightly. The dumbbells will lower to about knee height.

PULL: In one continuous movement, explosively thrust your hips forward and stand up, rising up on your toes as you simultaneously shrug your shoulders, bend your elbows, and pull the dumbbells up to shoulder height. Lower the dumbbells to the Setup position and repeat.

PERFORMANCE POINTER

PUSH THEN PULL.
Push your hips forward before shrugging your shoulders. The hip snap starts the dumbbells moving explosively; from there, the movement should be fluid as you simultaneously pull up your elbows and explosively jump onto your toes.

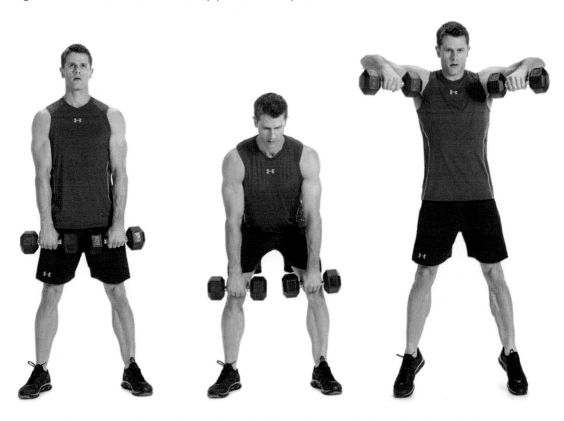

SNATCH

TARGET MUSCLES: total body

SETUP: Stand with your feet slightly wider than shoulder-width apart and a dumbbell resting on the floor between your feet, ends facing to the sides. Squat down and grab the dumbbell with your right hand, palm facing back. Your left arm should hang down at your side.

PULL: In one continuous—and explosive—motion, drive your heels into the floor and straighten your legs and hips while simultaneously bending your right arm and raising your elbow as high as possible to pull the dumbbell upward. (Imagine you're trying to thrust the dumbbell up toward the ceiling without letting go of it.)

As the dumbbell reaches chest level, let your forearm rotate up and back from the momentum of the lift as you push your hips forward and drop into a shallow squat to "catch" the dumbbell above you. While squatting and catching, straighten your arm and your legs. At the top, you should be in a standing position with the dumbbell directly above your right shoulder, right arm straight, and palm facing forward. Reverse the motion to bring the dumbbell back into the Setup position, and repeat. Perform the required number of repetitions, switch sides, and repeat.

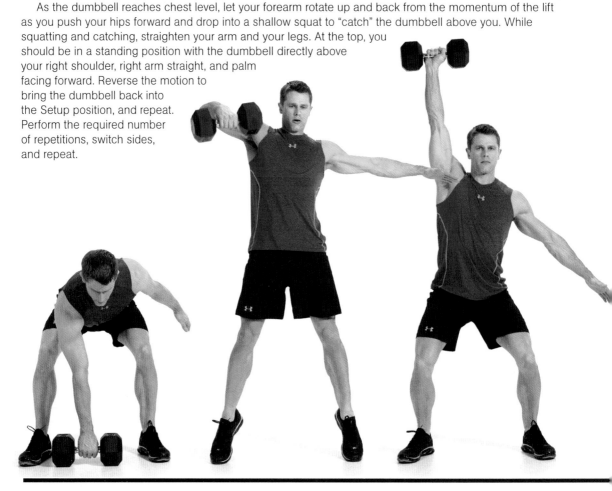

Other Dumbbell Exercises to Try

The following exercises shown in the kettlebell chapter (see page 89) can also be performed with a dumbbell or dumbbells.

- ▶ 45-Degree Two-Arm Row (page 99)
- ▶ Yates Row (page 99)
- ▶ Bent Press (page 101)
- ▶ Farmer's Walk (page 102)

- ▶ Swings (pages 106 and 108)
- ▶ High Pull (page 112)
- ▶ Iron Cross (page 117)
- ▶ Sots Press (page 121)
- ▶ Goblet Lunge (page 123)
- ▶ Goblet Squat (page 126)
- ▶ Renegade Row (page 130)
- ▶ Turkish Getup (page 132)
- ▶ Half Getup (page 133)
- ▶ Windmill (page 134)

The following exercise in the sandbag chapter can be performed with dumbbells:

- ▶ Bottom-Half Getup (page 165)

PERFORMANCE POINTERS

STAY TIGHT.
Keep the dumbbell as close to your body as possible at all times. Pulling up while it's away from your body may put undue strain on your shoulder and lower back.

USE ENOUGH POWER.
The force of your pull upward should make you rise up on your toes.

THINK "ARM TO EAR."
Concentrate on the position of your arm at the top. It should line up just behind your ear. Positioning it too far behind your head can hyperextend your lower back.

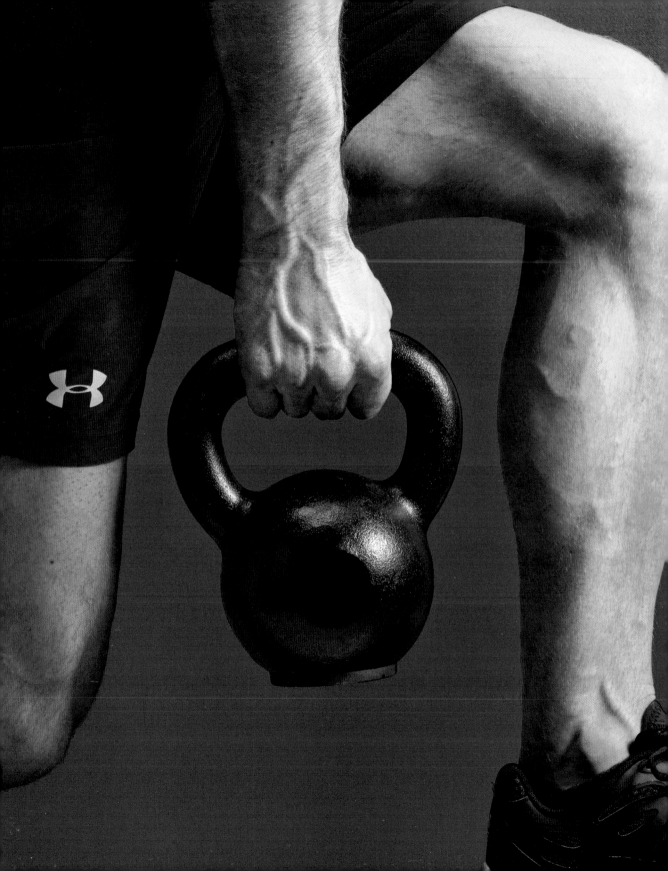

THE BEST KETTLEBELL EXERCISES

PUSH, PULL, SWING WITH THIS
NO-NONSENSE WORK CAPACITY TOOL

Kettlebells work for bodybuilding because they are so mechanically unwieldy. They're awkward, heavy, and difficult to balance, so they challenge your muscles in unique ways.

Before you use one of these weights, jump to Chapter 9 and take a kettlebell for a test drive to build muscular familiarity with the tool. In addition, learn how to "rack" a kettlebell. This is a technique used in Overhead Presses, Lunges, and Squats. To rack, raise the kettlebell in front of your shoulders with the round part (the bell) resting in the crook of your elbow and your elbow pointing directly toward your hip. To do this, you have two options: If the weight is light enough that you can curl it into position by your shoulders, do that. If the weight is too heavy, or you just want to get a little extra benefit from raising the weight into position, the smartest way is to clean the kettlebell to your shoulder. That move is a good place to start our review of killer kettlebell exercises.

CLEAN

TARGET MUSCLES: back, chest, core, glutes, hamstrings, and quadriceps

SETUP: Stand tall with your feet hip-width apart and hold a kettlebell with your right hand with an overhand grip, palm facing behind you. Unlock your knees, push your hips back, and lean forward at your waist. (Your knees will bend slightly as you go.) Your right arm should hang straight down in front of you, between your legs, palm facing back, and your left arm can hang at your side.

PULL: In one move, swing the weight back between your legs, then quickly push yourself up into a standing position by squeezing your glutes, thrusting your hips forward, and pushing your feet into the floor. Simultaneously swing the kettlebell up toward your right shoulder and "catch" it. The kettlebell should be resting along the back of your forearm up by your shoulder, with the bell "racked" or resting in the crook of your right elbow. Now the kettlebell is positioned where you need it to be in order to perform whatever exercise you'll be doing.

However, if the exercise you're looking to do is an actual Kettlebell Clean, then simply reverse the motion to get back into the Setup position. Perform the required number of repetitions, switch sides, and repeat.

PERFORMANCE POINTERS

LEAVE YOUR BICEPS OUT.
If your arms are curling even a portion of the weight up, you're not allowing your hips to do their job.

WIGGLE YOUR TOES.
Keep your feet flat at the start, but make sure you can wiggle your toes. That will tell you that the weight is loaded more along the back of your body.

DON'T BEND YOUR WRIST.
Your knuckles should be in line with your wrist and elbow at the top. Don't let the weight of the kettlebell bend your wrist backward.

OPTIONS

DOUBLE CLEAN
Take a slightly wider than shoulder-width stance, and hold a kettlebell in each hand. Perform the exercise as explained at left.

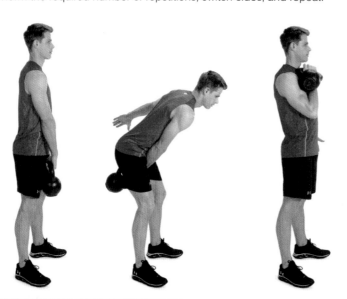

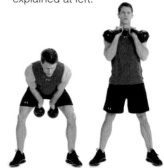

HANG CLEAN

Perform the exercise as explained on the opposite page, but don't swing the kettlebell through your legs to begin the lift. This will remove some momentum from the move, making it harder to pull the kettlebell.

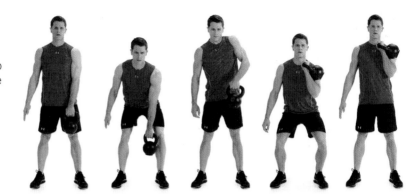

DEAD CLEAN

Perform the exercise as explained in the Hang Clean, but begin with the bell resting on the floor directly in front of you.

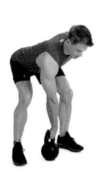
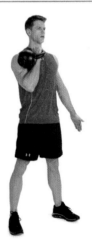

SAVE YOUR FOREARMS

When performing Kettlebell Cleans (and other exercises, such as the Kettlebell Snatch), the bell naturally changes position by flipping over your fist as you swing it up to either your shoulder or above your head. A common problem is that if you don't get under the bell and let it rotate over your hands in the right way, the bell can swing down with force and smash against the back of your forearm. To avoid this, keep a loose (but steady) grip on the kettlebell; as it rises to your shoulder, quickly rotate your hand and punch upward to make the bell rotate around without slamming into your arm.

CLEAN AND PRESS

TARGET MUSCLES: back, chest, core, glutes, hamstrings, quadriceps, shoulders, and triceps

SETUP: Stand holding a kettlebell with your left hand with an overhand grip, palm facing behind you. Unlock your knees, push your hips back, and lean forward at your waist. (Your knees will bend slightly as you go.) Your left arm should hang straight down in front of you between your legs, palms facing back, and your right arm can hang at your side.

PULL AND PUSH: In one move, swing the weight back between your legs, then quickly push yourself up into a standing position by squeezing your glutes, thrusting your hips forward, and pushing your feet into the floor. Simultaneously swing the kettlebell up toward your left shoulder.

If the kettlebell is very heavy, right before it reaches your left shoulder, quickly drop into a slight squat (not shown) and get your elbow underneath the kettlebell to rack it. Dip down a few inches by bending your knees, then quickly push the kettlebell up over your head as you push through your heels. Reverse the motion to lower the kettlebell back down into the Setup position, and repeat.

KEEP YOUR FEET FLAT.
Be sure you can wiggle your toes. That will tell you that the weight is loaded more along the back of your body.

DIP A LITTLE.
Getting under the kettlebell as it flips over your wrist and lands on your forearm at the top helps you absorb the impact.

KEEP YOUR WRIST STRAIGHT.
Your knuckles should be in line with your wrist and elbow at the top. Don't let the weight of the kettlebell bend your wrist backward.

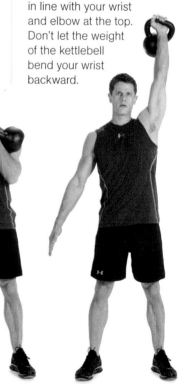

OPTION

DOUBLE CLEAN AND PRESS

Take a slightly wider than shoulder-width stance and hold a kettlebell in each hand. Perform the exercise as explained on the opposite page.

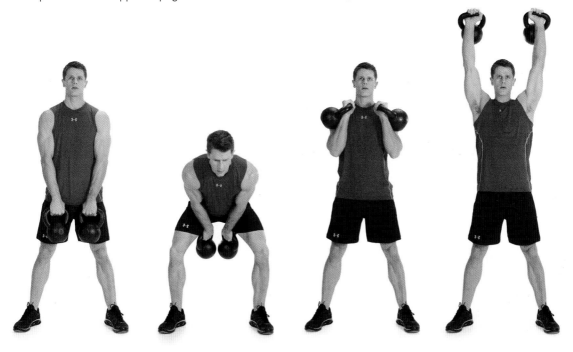

PLAY IT SAFE

For safety and greater stability, wear flat-soled workout shoes instead of running or cross-training shoes. Practice in front of a mirror so you can master the proper form. Exercise on a rubber workout mat or outdoors on grass, in case you have to drop the kettlebell.

AROUND-THE-BODY PASS

TARGET MUSCLES: back, core, and shoulders

SETUP: Stand with your feet shoulder-width apart and hold a kettlebell with both hands in front of your torso.

SWING: Contract your core muscles as you release the kettlebell into your right hand and move both arms behind your back. Grab the bell with your left hand, bring it back to the front (completing a full circle around your body), and repeat.

PERFORMANCE POINTERS

GO IN BOTH DIRECTIONS. Try to evenly divide passing the kettlebell clockwise and counterclockwise, instead of moving the kettlebell in the same direction all of the time.

MINIMIZE YOUR MOVEMENTS. For maximum results, avoid moving your hips as you perform the exercise.

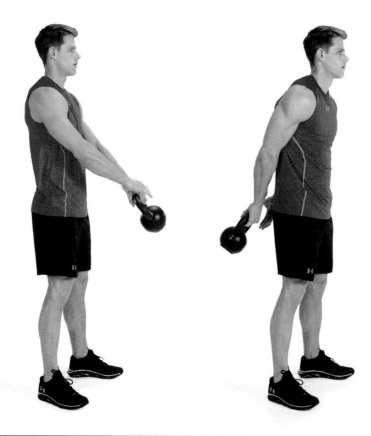

OPTION

AROUND-THE-LEGS PASS

With your feet less than hip-width apart and your arms hanging down in front of you, bend your knees until the bell is at about shin height. Contract your core muscles as you pass the bell around your legs. After half of the required reps, switch directions.

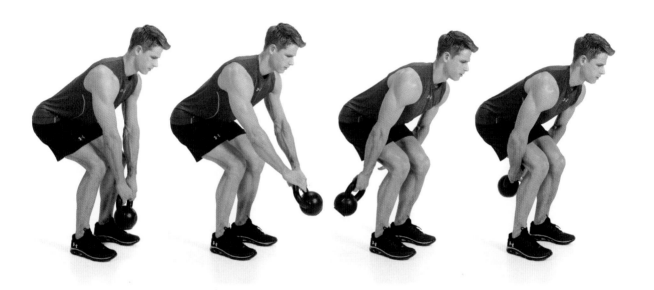

DID YOU KNOW?

Blueberries may aid in burning belly fat, according to the University of Michigan Cardiovascular Center. In a study conducted by researchers at the university, rats consuming only 2 percent of their diet in blueberries significantly reduced their abdominal fat within 90 days, as well as lowered triglyceride levels and increased insulin sensitivity. These results are thought to be a result of the high percentage of antioxidants—agents that rid the body of toxins—that occur naturally in blueberries.

FIGURE-EIGHT

TARGET MUSCLES: back, core, glutes, hamstrings, and quadriceps

SETUP: Stand with your feet wider than shoulder-width apart and place a kettlebell between your feet. Push your hips back, sink down into a half-squat (about halfway between a standing position and having your thighs parallel to the floor), and grab the kettlebell with your left hand.

SWING: Keeping your legs fixed in this position, you're going to pass the kettlebell back and forth between your legs. Use your left arm to gently swing the kettlebell underneath your body and toward your right knee as you simultaneously reach behind your right knee with your right hand and grab the kettlebell. Swing the kettlebell out, around, and back through your legs, toward your left knee. Grab it from behind your left knee with your left hand, and repeat.

PERFORMANCE POINTER

GO IN BOTH DIRECTIONS. Try to evenly divide passing the kettlebell clockwise and counterclockwise, instead of moving the kettlebell in the same figure-eight direction all the time.

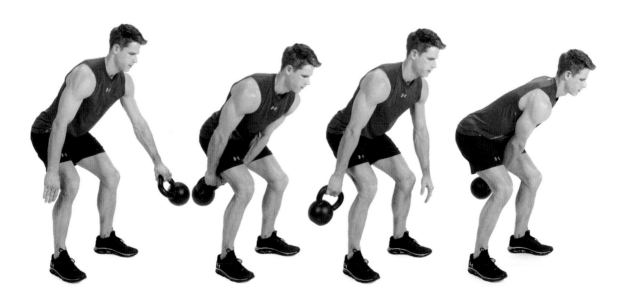

DEADLIFT

TARGET MUSCLES: trapezius, lower back, quadriceps, hamstrings, glutes, calves, and abs

SETUP: Stand tall with your feet shoulder-width apart and a heavy kettlebell on the floor in front of your toes. Push your hips back, bend your knees, and grab the kettlebell with both hands with palms facing behind you.

PULL: With your chest up and back flat, slowly pull the kettlebell off the floor by standing up as you extend your hips forward. Pause, lower the kettlebell back down to the floor, and repeat.

PERFORMANCE POINTERS

DON'T LOOK DOWN.
Looking at the kettlebell will cause your lower back to round.

KEEP YOUR ARMS STRAIGHT.
Resist the urge to raise your shoulders or bend your elbows as you go. Your shoulders should remain pulled back and down at the top of the lift, and the kettlebell should stay close to your body until your legs are straight but not locked.

OPTION

DOUBLE DEADLIFT
Grab a kettlebell in each hand and perform the exercise as explained.

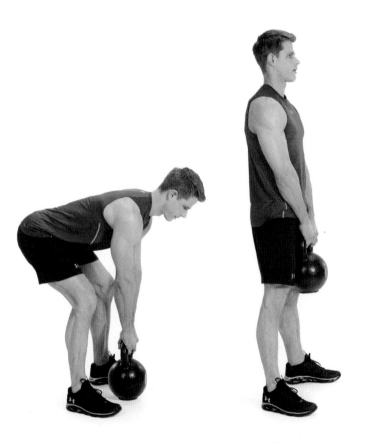

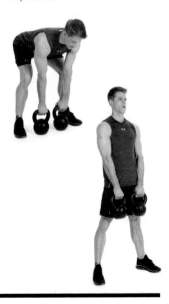

BENT-OVER ROW

TARGET MUSCLES: latissimus dorsi, lower back, middle trapezius, and rhomboids

SETUP: Stand tall in front of a bench with your feet hip-width apart, knees slightly bent, and a kettlebell in your right hand. Keeping your back flat, bend forward at your waist until your torso is almost parallel to the floor and support yourself by placing your left hand on the bench with a straight arm. Your right arm should extend straight down.

PULL: Without moving your upper body, pull the kettlebell up to the side of your torso. Pause, lower the kettlebell back down, and repeat. Perform the required reps, switch sides, and repeat.

PERFORMANCE POINTERS

KEEP NECK AND SPINE IN LINE. Lifting your head or turning your neck to see the kettlebell may strain your neck muscles. Instead, look down at the floor in front of you as you row.

MOVE ONLY YOUR ARM. Avoid twisting your torso and straightening your legs in order to lift the kettlebell, which is cheating.

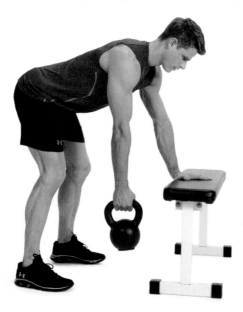

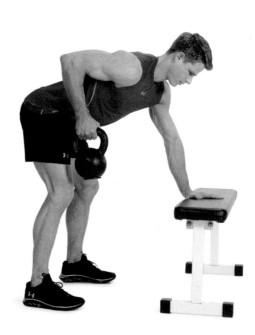

OPTIONS

45-DEGREE TWO-ARM ROW

Hold kettlebells in both hands and bend at the waist until your torso is 45 degrees to the floor. Pull the kettlebells to your sides and squeeze your shoulderblades together.

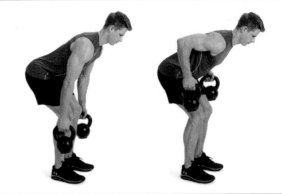

YATES ROW

Perform the exercise as explained on the opposite page, but only lower your torso 20 to 25 degrees and turn your wrists so your palms face forward.

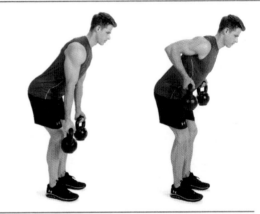

SINGLE-LEG ROW

With a light kettlebell in each hand, bend your left knee to raise your right foot off the floor and toward your butt, then slowly bend forward at your waist until your back is almost parallel to the floor, letting your arms hang straight down below you. Perform the exercise as explained on the opposite page.

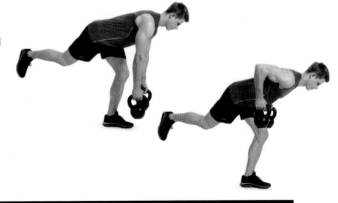

ROMANIAN DEADLIFT

TARGET MUSCLES: back, glutes, and hamstrings

SETUP: Stand tall with your feet shoulder-width apart and knees slightly bent. Hold a kettlebell in each hand, arms hanging down in front of your legs, palms facing toward you.

PULL: Slowly push your hips back and sit back, allowing your knees to bend slightly as you allow the kettlebells to drop just below your knees, keeping your head and chest up as you go. Pull your torso back into the Setup position, and repeat.

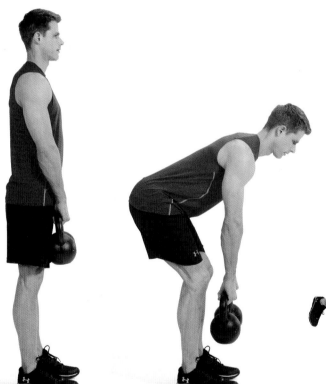

PERFORMANCE POINTER

DON'T SWING.
Keep the weights as close to your body as possible. This will focus all of the effort on your hamstrings, not your lower back.

OPTION

SINGLE-LEG ROMANIAN DEADLIFT

Holding a kettlebell in each hand, lift one foot behind you and hold it an inch or two off the floor so that you're balancing on the opposite foot. Holding this position, slowly shift your hips backward and bend forward until your back and rear leg are almost parallel to the floor. Let your arms hang straight down. Raise back up and repeat to perform the required number of reps. Afterward, switch sides and repeat.

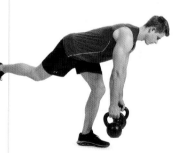

BENT PRESS

TARGET MUSCLES: total body, particularly the back, core, glutes, legs, and shoulders

SETUP: Stand tall with your feet shoulder-width apart, and hold a kettlebell in your right hand. Rack it by your right shoulder and let your left arm hang down at your side. Keeping your body facing forward, pivot your feet so that your toes point away from the weight at a 45-degree angle. Start pressing upward with your right hand to load the kettlebell behind your shoulder with your elbow pointing down and knuckles pointing up.

SWING: Although it's called a Press, the goal of this exercise is to keep the kettlebell suspended in place as you swing your torso down and away from the bell until your arm is straight. With your eyes on the kettlebell, keep the bell in place as you slowly push your hips to the right as far as possible, letting your left arm slide down your left leg toward the floor. Your right leg should stay straight as you go, but your left knee should bend to allow you to descend. As your torso lowers, your right arm will naturally straighten. Once your right arm is extended above you, stand back up. Once standing, lower the kettlebell to your shoulder, and repeat. Perform the required number of repetitions, switch sides, and repeat.

PERFORMANCE POINTERS

CONTRACT YOUR LATS.
This exercise relies a lot on your back muscles. Keeping them tight will help them do their job.

GO AS SLOWLY AS POSSIBLE.
Unlike many kettlebell exercises that require powerful, explosive movements, you'll see more results by moving in a slow, controlled fashion.

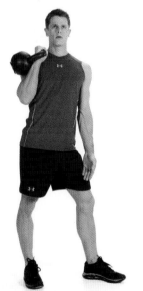 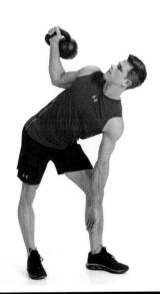 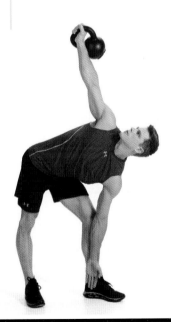

FARMER'S WALK

TARGET MUSCLES: calves, forearms, glutes, hamstrings, quadriceps, and traps

SETUP: Stand tall and grab a pair of heavy kettlebells, holding them as tightly as possible. Let your arms hang naturally at your sides, palms facing the sides of your legs, then pull your shoulders down and back while keeping your torso upright.

PUSH: Pushing off the balls of your feet, walk forward for the required distance or time.

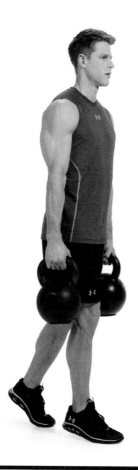

FOCUS ON YOUR FEET.
Paying attention to the weights may cause you to lift them by raising your shoulders, which can tire out your upper body before you thoroughly train your legs.

CHECK YOUR GRIP.
Wrap your thumbs over your fingers and squeeze. This exercise also improves grip strength.

BE SPACE SMART.
If you don't have enough room to walk, you can either walk in a circle or in a figure-eight pattern (both of which require far less space).

RAISE YOUR HEELS.
Balancing on the balls of your feet will shift extra effort onto your calf muscles.

OPTIONS

SUITCASE CARRY

Grab a heavy kettlebell in your nondominant hand and let it hang at arm's length next to your side. Let your other arm hang free. Brace your core and walk forward for the required time or distance (or as far as you can), keeping your chest up and torso straight. When finished, switch the kettlebell to your dominant hand and repeat.

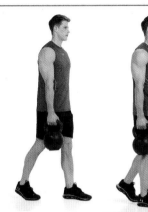

RACK WALK

Grab a pair of kettlebells lighter than you would usually use for the Farmer's Walk, rack them along your shoulders, and perform the exercise as explained on the opposite page.

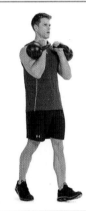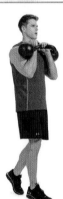

OVERHEAD FARMER'S WALK

Grab a pair of kettlebells lighter than you would usually use for the Farmer's Walk, then clean and push them over your head before you perform the exercise as explained on the opposite page.

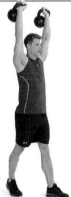

HIP HINGE AND STRETCHES

Performing a perfect Swing (as you'll learn on page 106) hinges on performing a Hip Hinge perfectly. The power that drives the kettlebell forward from between your legs is an explosive snap of your hips. For optimum benefit from a hip snap, it pays to put in the time practicing Hip Hinges and to stretch and strengthen your hips and core. The Wall Drill, Pushup-Position Plank, and hip stretches on these pages will help you get the most out of the highly metabolic Swing.

    Practice the Hip Hinge without a kettlebell until you have the movement perfected. The best way to practice is with an exercise called the Wall Drill.

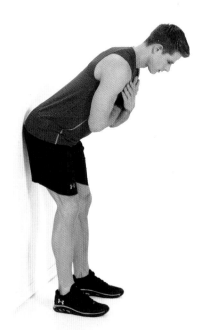

WALL DRILL

Stand with your back to a wall and your feet shoulder-width apart. Your heels should be about 6 inches from the wall. Keeping your legs mostly straight and your back straight, with a natural arch in your lower back, hinge at your hips until your butt touches the wall. Then straighten your body by pushing your hips forward. Step forward an inch or so and do another Hinge. Keep stepping, hinging, and touching the wall this way until you feel your hamstrings stretch and burn. That burning sensation in your hams indicates the perfect amount of hinge angle from which to perform the ideal hip snap for a kettlebell Swing. (It's sort of like a waiter's bow.) The stretch in your hams is like the tension in an archer's bow, and it delivers all the force you need to propel a kettlebell for perfect Swings. Practice it until it's immortalized in your muscle memory.

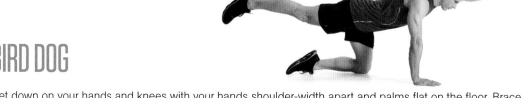

BIRD DOG

Get down on your hands and knees with your hands shoulder-width apart and palms flat on the floor. Brace your core and raise your left arm and right leg until they're in line with your torso. Hold for 5 to 10 seconds, and return to the starting position. Repeat with your right arm and left leg. Continue alternating arms and legs.

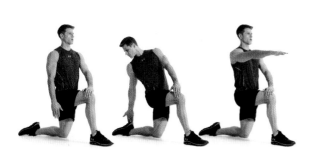

HIP FLEXOR RAINBOW

Assume a staggered stance, with your right foot 2 to 3 feet in front of your left and your feet hip-width apart. Lower your body until your left knee touches the floor and your right knee is bent at 90 degrees. Place your left hand on your right knee. This is the starting position. With your right hand, reach back as far as you can toward your toes. Keeping your right arm straight, arc your right hand over your head until it's straight out in front of your chest. Switch legs halfway through each set, unless otherwise indicated.

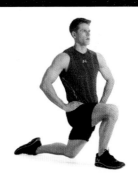

HIP FLEXOR STRETCH

Assume a staggered stance, with your right foot 2 to 3 feet in front of your left and your feet hip-width apart. This is the starting position. Lower your body until your left knee touches the floor and your right knee is bent at 90 degrees. Place both hands on your hips. Push your hips forward until you feel the stretch in your left hip and quad. Pause, and return to the starting position. Switch legs halfway through each set, unless otherwise indicated.

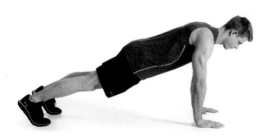

PUSHUP-POSITION PLANK

Assume a pushup position with your hands slightly beyond your shoulders and your arms and legs straight. Your body should form a straight line from your head to your ankles. Hold this position for the required amount of time.

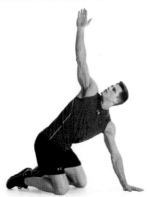

SIX-POINT ZENITH

Get down on your hands and knees. Keeping your back straight, twist your torso up to the right and swing your right arm toward the ceiling. Pause, and return to the starting position. Repeat with your left arm. Continue alternating sides.

SINGLE-ARM SWING

TARGET MUSCLES: back, core, glutes, and hamstrings

SETUP: Place a kettlebell on the floor in front of you. Stand with your feet slightly wider than shoulder-width apart, push your hips back as if shutting a door with your butt (your knees will bend slightly), and grab the kettlebell's handle with one hand. Your nonworking arm can hang at your side.

PULL: Keeping your back naturally arched, swing the weight between your legs and then squeeze your glutes and thrust your hips forward as you swing it to chest level. Swing the kettlebell back between your legs. That's 1 rep. Continue swinging for the required number of repetitions without returning to the starting position. Switch arms and repeat.

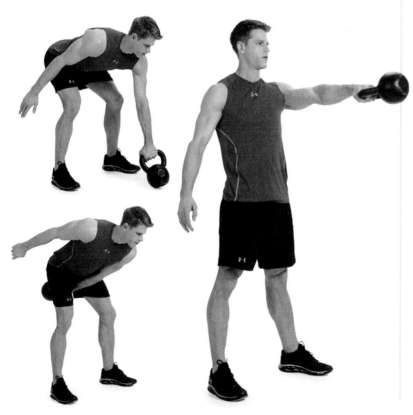

PERFORMANCE POINTERS

USE MOMENTUM.
Don't actively lift the kettlebell. But pull it back down between your legs consciously and under control.

USE YOUR HIPS.
Most men initiate the swing by squatting down and leaning forward, which can strain your back. Instead, perform a Hip Hinge. Push your hips back, keep your chest up, and maintain a natural arch in your lower back as you swing the kettlebell between your legs. (Practice with the Wall Drill on page 104.) Your forearms should touch your thighs, as if you were hiking a football.

KEEP PERFECT POSTURE.
To do this, imagine that the goal is to get your chin as far away from your tailbone as possible.

THINK HIPS NOT KNEES.
Minimize the bend in your knees. The swing is a Hip Hinge movement, not a squat. To get in the proper position, imagine you are at the start of performing a standing long jump.

STAY SHOULDER HEIGHT.
Never let the kettlebell go any higher than your head or you risk hyperextending your lower back.

OPTION

ALTERNATING SINGLE-ARM SWING

Keep both arms next to each other as you swing the kettlebell. At the top of the movement, right before the kettlebell begins to descend, switch the kettlebell to the opposite hand. Or switch hands at the bottom of the movement, when the bell is between your legs.

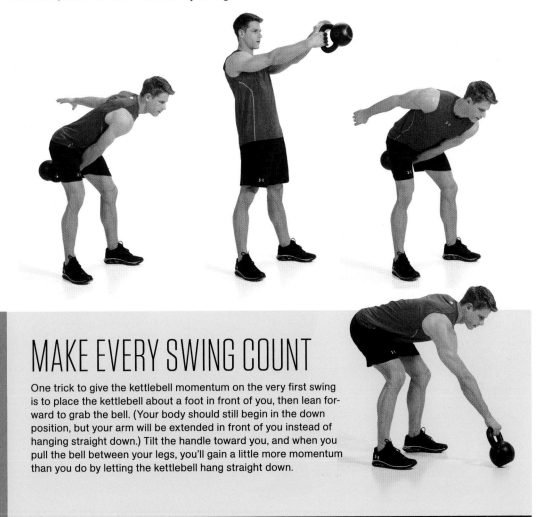

MAKE EVERY SWING COUNT

One trick to give the kettlebell momentum on the very first swing is to place the kettlebell about a foot in front of you, then lean forward to grab the bell. (Your body should still begin in the down position, but your arm will be extended in front of you instead of hanging straight down.) Tilt the handle toward you, and when you pull the bell between your legs, you'll gain a little more momentum than you do by letting the kettlebell hang straight down.

DOUBLE-ARM SWING

TARGET MUSCLES: back, core, glutes, legs, and shoulders

SETUP: Place a kettlebell on the floor in front of you. Stand with your feet slightly wider than shoulder-width apart, knees slightly bent, and grab the kettlebell with both hands. Perform a Hip Hinge by pushing your hips back as if trying to close a door with your butt, and lean forward at your waist.

PULL: Keeping your back naturally arched, swing the weight between your legs and then thrust your hips forward as you swing it to chest level. Swing it back between your legs. That's 1 rep. Continue swinging without returning to the starting position.

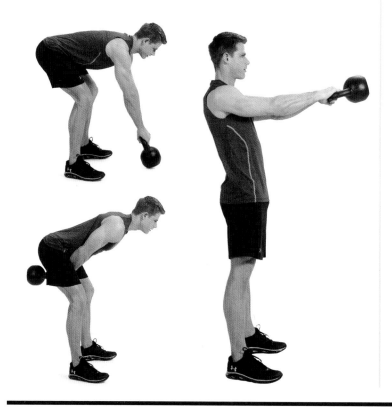

USE YOUR HIPS.
Most men initiate the swing by squatting down and leaning forward, which can strain your back. Instead, perform a Hip Hinge. Push your hips back, keep your chest up, and maintain a natural arch in your lower back as you swing the kettlebell between your legs. (Practice with the Wall Drill on page 104.)

KEEP PERFECT POSTURE.
Keep your shoulders back and in line. The weight shouldn't pull you. To do this, imagine that the goal is to get your chin as far away from your tailbone as possible.

MINIMIZE THE KNEE BEND.
The swing is a Hip Hinge movement, not a squat. To get in the proper position, imagine you are at the start of performing a standing long jump.

OPTIONS

WALKING SWING

Perform the exercise as explained on the opposite page, but raise the kettlebell to eye level. Just as the kettlebell reaches its highest point, quickly take a small step forward with *each foot* and realign your feet before the bell swings between your legs. Keep moving forward one small step per swing.

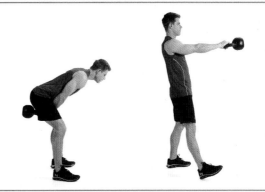

HALF-TURN SWING

Perform the exercise as explained on the opposite page, but pull the kettlebell higher to buy enough time to step in a half circle so that you're facing the opposite direction. Continue to turn yourself around 180 degrees with every swing.

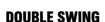

DOUBLE SWING

Grab a kettlebell in each hand and take a wider than shoulder-width stance. Perform the exercise as explained on the opposite page, but start with small swings to make sure you have enough distance between your legs to clear both kettlebells.

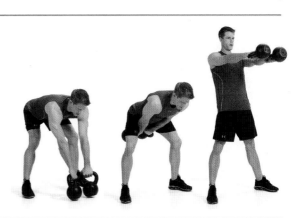

SNATCH

TARGET MUSCLES: total body

SETUP: Stand holding a kettlebell with your right hand with an overhand grip. Unlock your knees, push your hips back, and lean forward at your waist. (Your knees will bend slightly as you go.) Your right arm should hang straight down in front of you, between your legs, palm facing back. Your left arm can hang at your side.

PULL, SWING, AND PUSH: In one move, swing the weight back between your legs, then in one continuous and explosive motion, drive your heels into the floor and straighten your legs and hips while simultaneously swinging the kettlebell upward. (Imagine you're trying to thrust the kettlebell up toward the ceiling without letting go of it.)

As the kettlebell reaches eye level, flip it over so the bell is against your forearm as you push it overhead. At the top, you should be in a standing position with the kettlebell directly above your right shoulder, right arm straight, palm facing forward. Reverse the motion to bring the kettlebell back into the Setup position, and repeat. Perform the required number of repetitions, switch sides, and repeat.

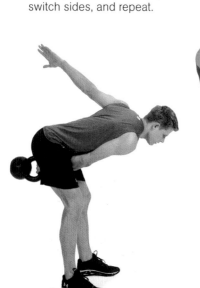
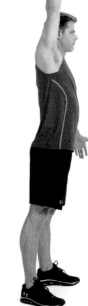

PERFORMANCE POINTERS

WATCH YOUR WRIST.
Don't let the kettlebell turn over and smack your wrist. You want to move your hand "around" the bell.

THINK "J" NOT ARC.
By tracing the path of the weight as a "J," you will keep the kettlebell close to your body as it rises, which will reduce the strain on your shoulder.

USE ENOUGH POWER.
If using a heavy kettlebell, pull up with enough force so that you rise onto your toes in the top position.

CONCENTRATE ON THE TOP.
Your arm should line up just behind your ear. Positioning it too far behind your head can hyperextend your lower back.

OPTION

TWO-HAND SNATCH

Hold a kettlebell in each hand and perform the exercise as explained on the opposite page.

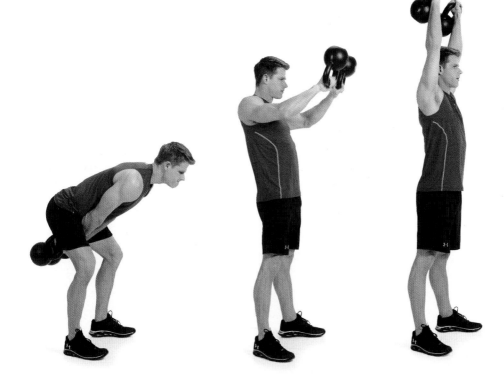

THE BEST KETTLEBELL EXERCISES

HIGH PULL

TARGET MUSCLES: biceps, calves, core, glutes, hamstrings, posterior deltoids, quadriceps, and upper and lower back

SETUP: Stand with your feet shoulder-width apart and a kettlebell on the floor in front of you. Push your hips back and squat down to grab the kettlebell with both hands, palms facing in.

PULL: In one continuous movement, explosively thrust your hips forward and pull the kettlebell off the floor, rising up on your toes as you simultaneously shrug your shoulders, bend your elbows, and pull the kettlebell up to shoulder height. Lower the kettlebell back down to the floor, return to the Setup position, and repeat.

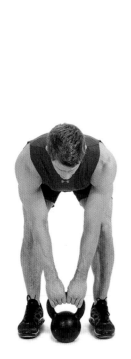
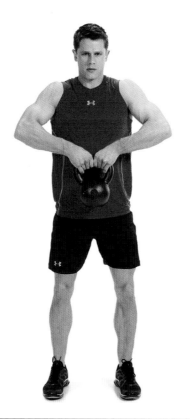
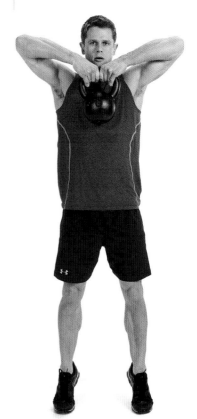

OPTIONS

DOUBLE HIGH PULL

Grab a lighter kettlebell with each hand and perform the exercise as explained on the opposite page.

ONE-ARM HIGH PULL

Grab a kettlebell with one hand and pull it up to your working arm's shoulder. Perform the required number of repetitions, switch sides, and repeat.

PUSHUP

TARGET MUSCLES: chest, core, shoulders, and triceps

SETUP: Kneel on the floor with two kettlebells in front of you, spaced about shoulder-width apart. Grab the kettlebells and get into a pushup position. (Note: Make sure the kettlebells are large enough that their bases can support you without tipping over.) Your arms should be straight, palms facing in. Your legs should be extended behind you, feet close together.

PUSH: Bend your elbows and lower your chest down toward the floor. Push yourself back up until your arms are straight but not locked, and repeat.

PERFORMANCE POINTERS

WATCH YOUR POSTURE.
Your body should form a straight line from your head down to your heels, and your eyes should be focused on the floor.

KEEP YOUR ELBOWS IN.
Winging them out redirects the stress of the move to your elbow joints.

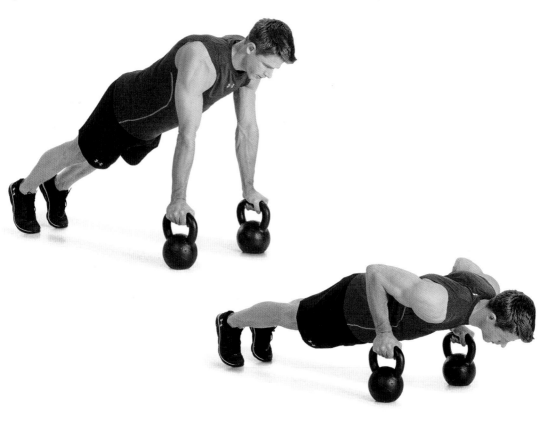

PUSHUP DRAG

Start in a pushup position with a kettlebell on the floor next to your left side. Bend your elbows, lower your chest toward the floor, then push yourself back up until your arms are straight. Shift your weight to your left arm as you reach your right arm underneath your body to grab the kettlebell. Drag it underneath you with your right hand until it rests at your right side. Do another Pushup and repeat, this time using your left hand to drag the weight to your left side.
Extra credit: Includes a Swing!

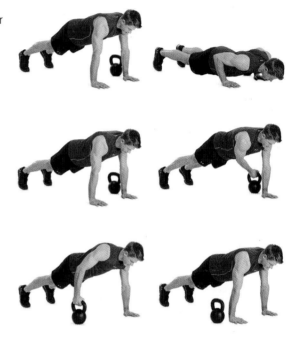

DEATH CRAWL

Perform one Pushup on kettlebells, then balance on your left arm and row the kettlebell in your right hand up to your side. When you lower it to the floor, place the kettlebell in line with your shoulder but a few inches ahead of where you started. Do another Pushup, then row the kettlebell in your left hand, placing it back down a few inches ahead of your right hand. Continue to "crawl" forward by doing one Pushup and one Row.

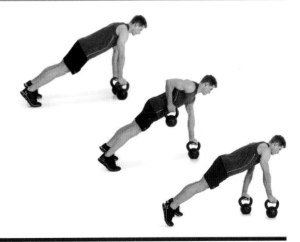

HALO

TARGET MUSCLES: back, shoulders, triceps, and core

SETUP: Grab a light kettlebell by the handle with both hands, bell end facing up, and hold it in front of your chest with your elbows bent.

SWING: Raise the kettlebell up and circle it clockwise around your head. After half of the required reps, switch directions.

PERFORMANCE POINTERS

BRACE YOUR CORE.
Don't let the momentum of the move pull your torso to the side. Minimizing your side-to-side movements will mean you're engaging more of your core.

WATCH YOUR WRISTS.
The kettlebell should be heavy enough to be a challenge, but not so heavy that it's difficult to keep your wrists from bending.

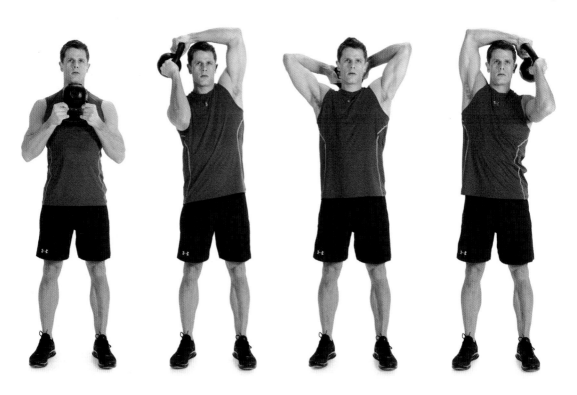

IRON CROSS

TARGET MUSCLES: shoulders and upper trapezius

SETUP: Stand tall with your feet shoulder-width apart and hold a kettle-bell in each hand. Rack them by your shoulders, then push the kettle-bells up over your shoulders until your arms are straight, palms facing forward. Keep your elbows close to the sides of your head.

PULL: Keeping your arms straight, slowly lower the kettlebells out to your sides until your arms are parallel to the floor—your body should look like a T. Pause, then pull your arms back into the Setup position, and repeat.

PERFORMANCE POINTERS

KEEP YOUR ARMS IN LINE. Don't let them stray too far forward or backward.

SQUEEZE YOUR GLUTES. Once the kettlebells are over your head, squeezing your glutes forces your body into a position that automatically stabilizes your spine.

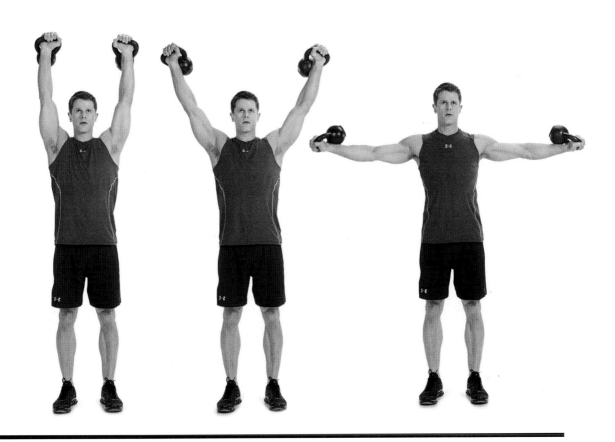

SHOULDER PRESS

TARGET MUSCLES: shoulders, triceps, and upper trapezius

SETUP: Stand tall with your feet shoulder-width apart, and hold a kettlebell in your right hand. Rack it by your right shoulder so the bell is resting along the back of your forearm. Your left arm can either hang at your side or you can place your left hand on your hip.

PUSH: With your back straight and eyes looking forward, push the weight up over your head until your arm is straight and your elbow is locked. Lower the kettlebell back down to your shoulder and repeat. Perform the required number of repetitions, switch sides, and repeat.

PERFORMANCE POINTERS

SQUEEZE YOUR GLUTES.
Once the kettlebell is over your head, squeezing your glutes forces your body into a position that automatically stabilizes your spine.

TAKE A KNEE.
The Shoulder Press and its variations can also be done from a kneeling position.

BRACE YOUR CORE.
Tightening your stomach as if you could get hit at any time will further stabilize your body.

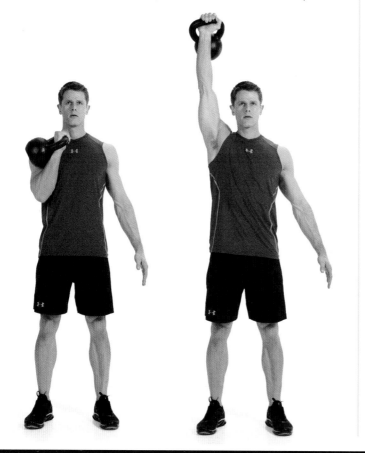

OTHER OPTIONS

TWO-HAND SHOULDER PRESS

Hold a kettlebell in each hand and press both up at the same time.

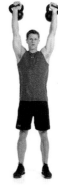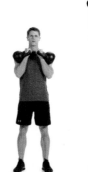

SEESAW PRESS

Hold a kettlebell in each hand. Press one bell up as you lower the other bell. Alternate in seesaw fashion with control. ***Extra credit: Includes a Swing!***

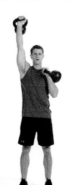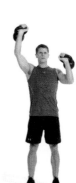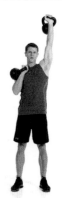

BOTTOM-UP SHOULDER PRESS

Perform the exercise as explained on the opposite page, but hold the kettlebell so that the bell is directly over the handle the entire time.

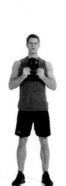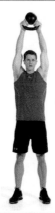

SINGLE-ARM PUSH PRESS

TARGET MUSCLES: shoulders, triceps, upper trapezius, core, and legs

SETUP: Stand tall with your feet shoulder-width apart, and hold a kettlebell in your right hand. Rack it by your right shoulder so it is resting on the outside of your forearm with your palm facing in, and let your left arm hang straight down at your side.

PUSH: Keeping your back straight and eyes looking forward, squat down about 6 inches, look up, then explosively push up with your legs as you push the kettlebell straight above your right shoulder. Pause, slowly lower yourself and the kettlebell back into the Setup position, and repeat. Perform the required number of repetitions, switch sides, and repeat.

PERFORMANCE POINTER

PUSH THROUGH YOUR HEELS. This will give you more power when pushing the kettlebell directly overhead.

OPTION

TWO-ARM PUSH PRESS

Grab a single kettlebell in each hand and perform the exercise as explained.

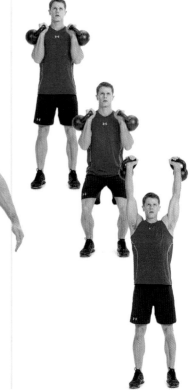

SOTS PRESS

TARGET MUSCLES: glutes, hamstrings, quadriceps, shoulders, triceps, core, and upper back

SETUP: Stand tall with your feet shoulder-width apart, and hold a kettlebell in your right hand. Rack it by your right shoulder and let your left arm hang at your side. Push your hips back and sink into a deep squat.

PUSH: Holding yourself in the squat, press the kettlebell overhead until your right arm is locked straight above your right shoulder. Next, lower the kettlebell into the Setup position, and repeat. Perform the required number of repetitions, stand up, switch sides, and repeat.

PERFORMANCE POINTERS

RECOGNIZE YOUR LIMITS.
If you can't sink down into a full squat to start, do the exercise from a quarter- or half-squat position (as shown) and try to go lower each time you perform it.

KEEP YOUR CORE TIGHT.
Push down through your heels and contract your midsection to give yourself enough stability and power.

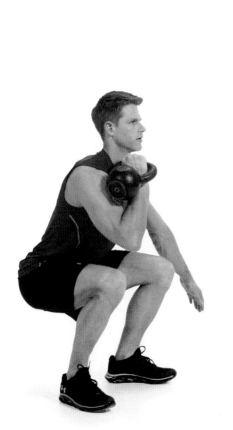
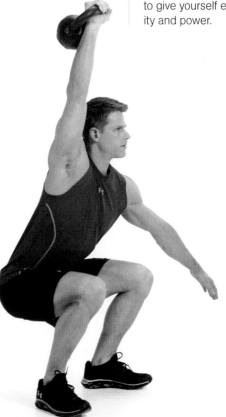

REVERSE LUNGE

TARGET MUSCLES: calves, core, glutes, hamstrings, and quadriceps

SETUP: Stand tall with your feet hip-width apart, and hold a kettlebell in each hand. Rack the kettlebells by your shoulders so that they are resting on your forearms.

PUSH: Take a big step backward with your right foot and lower yourself by bending your left knee until your left thigh is parallel to the floor. Pause, push yourself back up into the Setup position, then step back with your left leg. Pause and push yourself back into the Setup position. That's 1 rep.

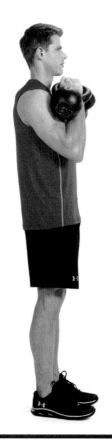
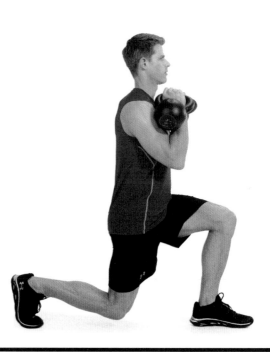

OPTIONS

OVERHEAD LUNGE

Push the kettlebells over your head first, then perform the exercise as explained on the opposite page.

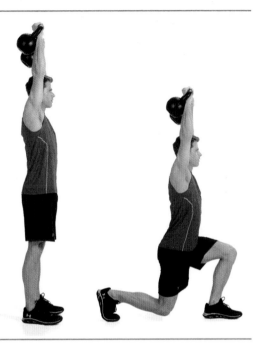

GOBLET LUNGE

Use both hands to hold a heavy kettlebell vertically against your chest, cupping the kettlebell head like a goblet, elbows pointing toward the floor. Perform the exercise as explained on the opposite page.

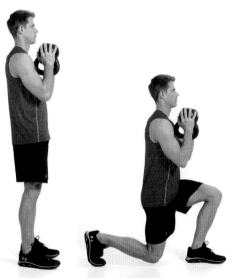

TACTICAL LUNGE

TARGET MUSCLES: quadriceps, hamstrings, glutes, and calves

SETUP: Stand tall with your feet hip-width apart and a kettlebell in your right hand. Your arms should be hanging at your sides, palms facing in.

PUSH AND SWING: Take a big step backward with your right foot and bend your left knee until your left thigh is parallel to the floor. In this Lunge position, pass the kettlebell from your right hand to your left hand underneath your left leg.

Push yourself back up into the Setup position, then step back with your left leg and bend your right knee until your right thigh is parallel to the floor. Pass the kettlebell from your left hand to your right hand. That's 1 repetition.

PERFORMANCE POINTER

KEEP YOUR BACK UPRIGHT. As the kettlebell passes underneath your leg, you may feel the urge to look down. Don't. Instead, keep your back flat and your chest up.

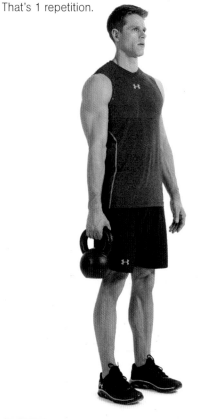
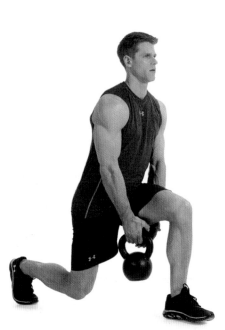

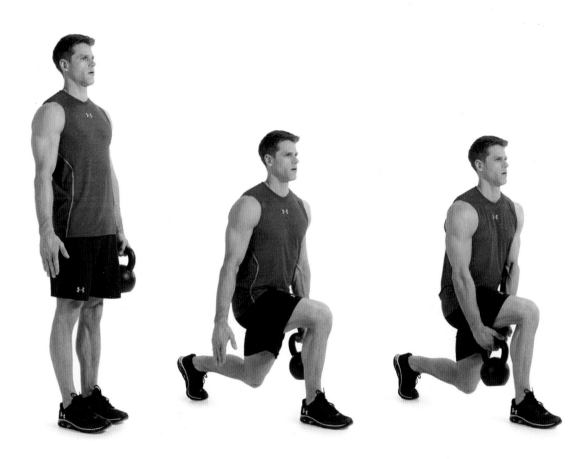

GOBLET SQUAT

TARGET MUSCLES: glutes, hamstrings, quadriceps, and calves

SETUP: Stand tall with your feet shoulder-width apart and hold a heavy kettlebell with both hands in front of your chest. You can either cup the bottom of the kettlebell with your palms or you can grab the sides of the handle.

PUSH: Keeping your torso straight, chest up, and the kettlebell held in front of you, push your hips back, bend your knees, and squat down as far as you can, past the point where your thighs are parallel with the floor. Pause at the bottom, explode back up into the Setup position, and repeat.

PERFORMANCE POINTERS

CHOOSE THE RIGHT WEIGHT. A kettlebell that's too heavy to hold may tire out your arms before your legs get a thorough workout. Instead of going too heavy, pick a kettlebell that you are able to manage without having to quit too soon.

CONTRACT YOUR LATS. This trick gets your upper body more involved in the exercise.

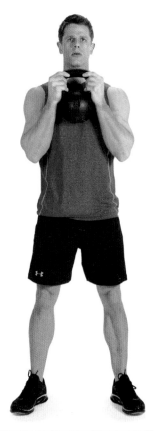
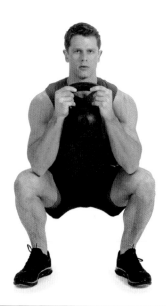

OPTIONS

WIDE-STANCE GOBLET SQUAT

Perform the exercise as explained on the opposite page, but space your feet about twice shoulder-width apart with your toes pointing out at an angle.

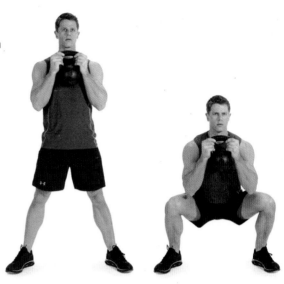

THRUSTER

Perform the exercise as explained on the opposite page, but as you stand back up, press the kettlebell over your head.

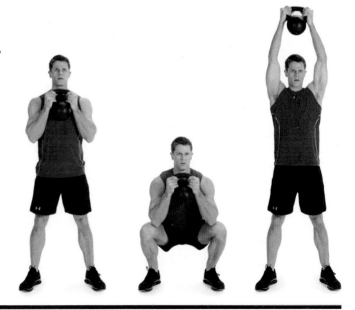

PISTOL SQUAT

TARGET MUSCLES: hip flexors, quadriceps, glutes, hamstrings, and core

SETUP: Stand on one leg with the other leg slightly extended in front of you. Hold a light kettlebell with both hands in front of your chest.

PUSH: Keeping your torso straight, chest up, and kettlebell in front of you, push your hips back and bend your knee to lower down slowly. Keep extending your elevated foot in front of you to keep it from touching the floor. Pause at the bottom, then extend your working leg to return to the starting position. Repeat the move on the same leg for the required reps before switching sides.

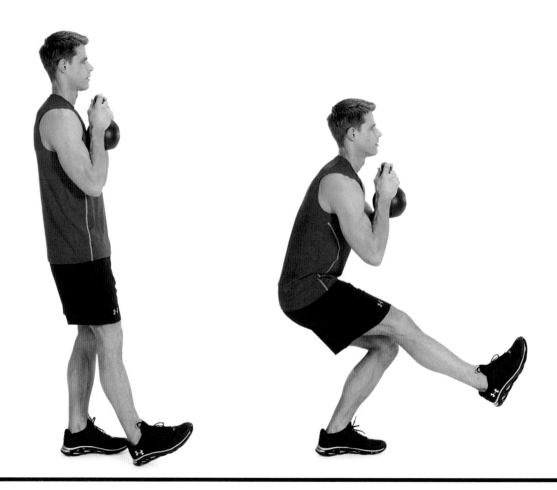

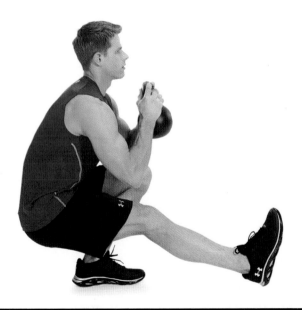

PERFORMANCE POINTERS

WATCH YOUR DEPTH.
Go as low as you can without overly rounding your lower back. Ideally, you want your extended leg to hover over the ground, but don't sacrifice your posture to reach that.

TRY IT SANS KETTLEBELL.
Practice performing the movement without a kettlebell and extend your arms straight in front of you instead (holding them there for the entire movement).

BEND YOUR ANKLE.
As you descend, the ankle of your working leg should bend so that your lower leg is angled, as opposed to remaining vertical (which is how your lower leg is positioned when performing a traditional squat).

STRETCH FIRST.
This move requires a great deal of hamstring flexibility to keep your nonworking leg extended straight in front of you and a lot of hip and ankle mobility.

RENEGADE ROW

TARGET MUSCLES: back, chest, core, shoulders, and triceps

SETUP: Kneel on the floor with two kettlebells in front of you, spaced 2 to 3 inches apart. Grab the kettlebells and get into a Pushup position. Your arms should be straight, palms facing in, elbows unlocked. Your legs should be extended behind you, feet hip- to shoulder-width apart.

PULL: Balancing yourself with your right arm, push down with your right hand as you slowly lift the kettlebell in your left hand off the floor and pull it toward your left side. Lower the kettlebell back to the floor, then repeat with your right arm. That's 1 rep.

PERFORMANCE POINTERS

GO BIG FOR SAFETY.
Make sure the kettlebells are large enough that their bases can support your weight without tipping over (12 kilograms is a good start).

HAVE HAPPY WRISTS.
You can experiment with spacing the kettlebells farther apart (but not more than shoulder-width apart) or turning the handles at an angle toward each other, so the tops of the handles make a backward V from overhead.

STAY BALANCED.
If the move is shaky with your feet hip-width apart, try spacing your feet shoulder-width apart, or even slightly wider.

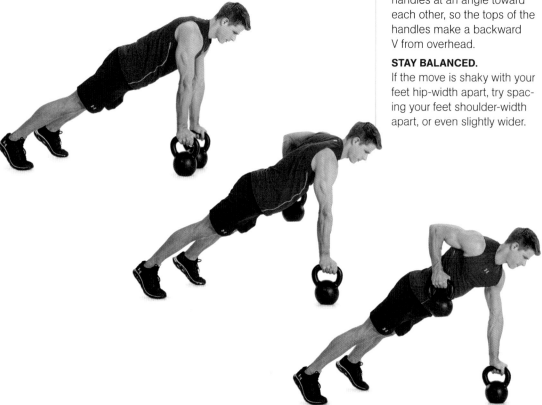

OPTION

RENEGADE ROW AND BURPEE

Perform the exercise as shown on the opposite page, but after one complete Renegade Row, continue to hold both kettlebells and quickly bring your legs toward your torso, feet right behind the kettlebells, then jump up. Once you land, squat, place the kettlebells back on the floor, kick your legs back into a Pushup position, and repeat.

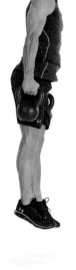

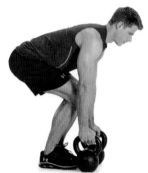

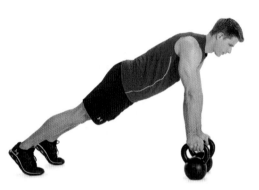

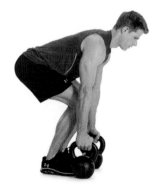

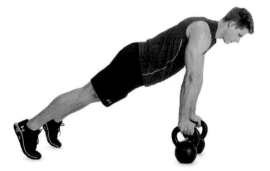

TURKISH GETUP

TARGET MUSCLES: core, glutes, hamstrings, lower back, and quadriceps

SETUP: Lie flat on your back holding a kettlebell in your left hand. Your right arm should extend at your side, palm flat on the floor. Straighten your left arm so that the weight is directly above you and the kettlebell rests against your forearm. Bend your left leg and place your left foot flat on the floor, and keep your right leg straight.

PUSH: Keeping your left elbow locked and the weight above you at all times, stand up in this sequence: Begin by rolling onto your right side to help prop yourself up on your right elbow, then push up with your right arm so you're resting on your right hand. Push yourself up into a half-kneel by threading your right leg behind your left leg. From there, begin to stand up, keeping the kettlebell above you at all times. Keeping your left arm straight, reverse the steps to return to the Setup position, then repeat. Perform the required number of repetitions, switch sides, and repeat.

PERFORMANCE POINTERS

KEEP YOUR EYE ON THE KETTLEBELL. Imagine that the goal of the entire move is to simply push the weight straight up toward the ceiling.

DON'T LIFT YOUR FOOT. Pushing the foot of your bent leg into the floor at all times will help you distribute the load more evenly and allow you to utilize more muscles, including your glutes and hips, which will give you more strength and power.

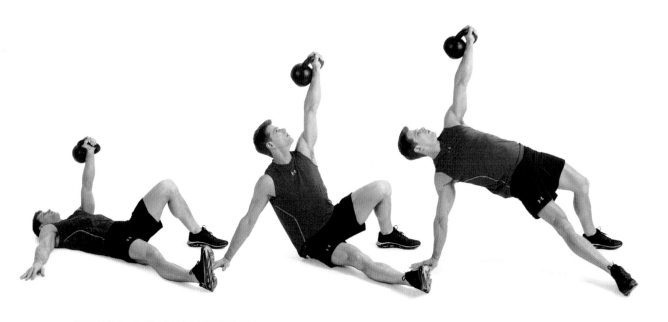

OPTION

HALF-GETUP

Lie on the floor, holding the kettlebell in your right hand straight above your shoulder. Bend your right knee, place your foot on the floor, and prop yourself up on your left elbow. Keep the weight directly in line with your shoulder, and sit up until your arm and back are straight. Reverse the movement to lie down. That's 1 rep. Complete all required reps, switch sides, and repeat.

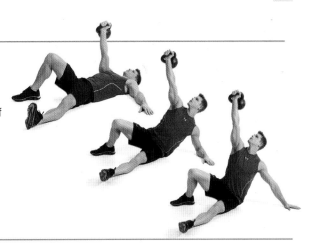

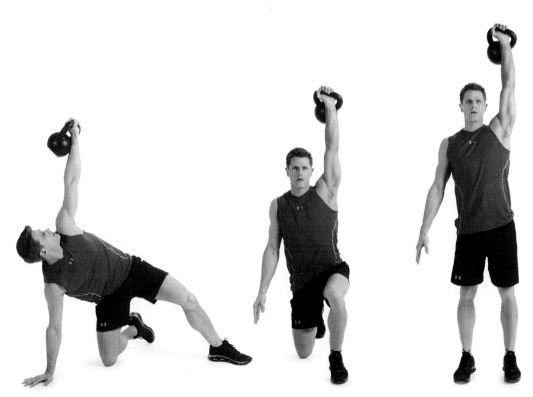

WINDMILL

TARGET MUSCLES: total body, particularly the core, glutes, hamstrings, and shoulders

SETUP: Stand tall with your feet slightly wider than shoulder-width apart and a light kettlebell in your right hand in front of your right shoulder, bell resting on the outside of your right arm. Push the weight overhead so that your right arm is straight and the kettlebell is directly above your right shoulder and resting on the back of your forearm. Keeping your body facing forward, pivot your feet so that your toes point to the left at a 45-degree angle.

SWING: With your right arm locked straight overhead and your eyes on the kettlebell, slowly shift your hips to the right as far as possible, letting your left arm slide down your left leg toward the floor. Your right leg should stay straight as you go, but your left knee should bend to allow you to descend. The goal is to touch the floor with your left hand.

Pause at the bottom, then quickly reverse the move to return to the Setup position and repeat. Perform the required number of repetitions, switch sides, and repeat.

MAINTAIN ALIGNMENT.
Your wrist should remain in line with your forearm and upper arm at all times.

KEEP YOUR CORE ENGAGED.
Don't let your spine flex from side to side or forward as you lower yourself.

PRACTICE WITHOUT WEIGHT.
To get the most out of the Windmill, form is key, so get your body used to the movement before adding a kettlebell.

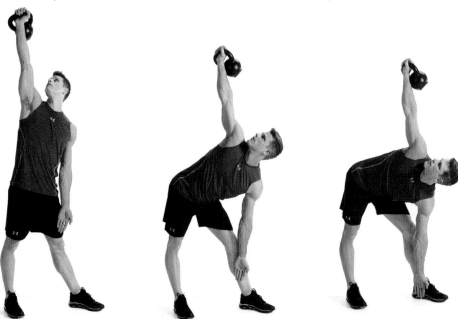

OPTION

DOUBLE WINDMILL

Hold a kettlebell in each hand. Once you've performed a Windmill with one arm, switch positions (and the angle of your feet) and perform another Windmill on the opposite side.

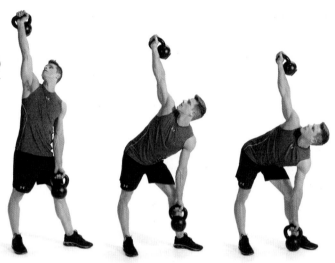

Other Kettlebell Exercises to Try

The following exercises, shown in the dumbbell chapter, also can be performed with one or two kettlebells.

- ▶ Biceps Curl (page 46)
- ▶ Chest Press (page 48)
- ▶ Chest Fly (page 50)
- ▶ Crunch (page 51)
- ▶ Front Squat (page 53)
- ▶ Squat (page 54)
- ▶ Straight-Leg Deadlift (page 59)
- ▶ Lateral Raise (page 60)
- ▶ Lunge (page 64)

- ▶ Side Lunge (page 65)
- ▶ Kneeling Twist (page 71)
- ▶ Standing Twist (page 73)
- ▶ Stepup (page 74)
- ▶ Lying Triceps Extension (page 80)
- ▶ Single-Arm Triceps Kickback (page 81)
- ▶ Overhead Triceps Extension (page 82)
- ▶ Pullover (page 83)

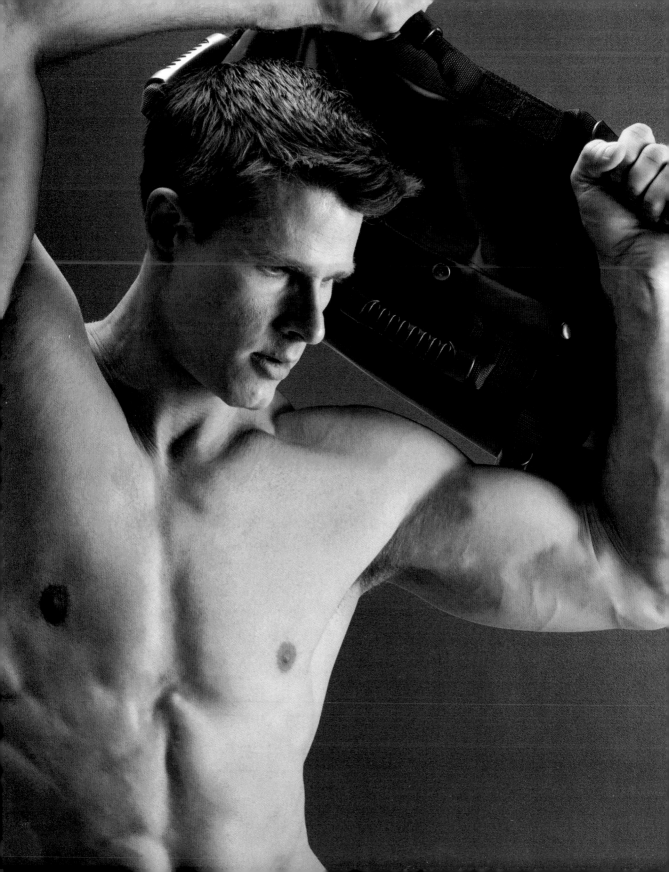

CHAPTER 8

THE BEST SANDBAG EXERCISES

PUSH, PULL, SWING FOR REAL-WORLD STRENGTH

Exercising with a sandbag harkens back to the days when men used their muscles to do a job, not a computer touchpad. We tossed bales of hay, stacked bags of grain, and swung pickaxes into coal. Sweating with a sandbag is just about as close as you can get to doing real work without getting paid. And there's really no better tool for functional exercise. The beauty of the sandbag is that the shifting grains of sand within the bag make the resistance unbalanced and ever changing, so your muscles keep having to adjust to maintain control and balance.

Since it's such an unstable piece of equipment, a little practice is helpful before you go full jarhead on this gear. Jump to Chapter 9 to familiarize yourself with the tool before tackling the exercises in this chapter. One more thing: Many sandbag exercises require a special way to hold the bag before initiating the main move. It's best to nail those before going forward, so let's begin there.

BEAR HUG

This setup move for many sandbag exercises is exactly what it sounds like. You grab the sandbag and hug it close to your chest.

TARGET MUSCLES: back, chest, core, glutes, legs, and shoulders

SETUP: Stand tall with your feet slightly wider than shoulder-width apart and toes pointing out at an angle. Position a sandbag vertically (with one end facing you) on the floor between your feet.

PULL: Keeping your low back arched, push your hips back, bend your knees, squat down, and scoop your fingers around both sides of the middle of the sandbag. Lift the sandbag off the floor and up against your chest by quickly pushing your hips forward, extending your knees, and squeezing your glutes. Simultaneously pull the sandbag up close to your chest, hugging it like a big (heavy) teddy bear. One end of the sandbag should be at about chin level, allowing you to see above it.

   To lower the sandbag, quickly reverse the motion by pushing your hips back and bending your knees. As you squat down, keep the sandbag close to your chest as you lower it back to the floor.

PERFORMANCE POINTER

SQUEEZE THE SANDBAG. Because this hold is one that's used as a Setup position for other sandbag exercises—such as the Bear Hug Squat and the Bear Hug Farmer's Walk—having a firm grip on the bag at all times is critical. Once you've hoisted the sandbag from the floor, take a second to get your arms farther around the sandbag so you have more control of the weight.

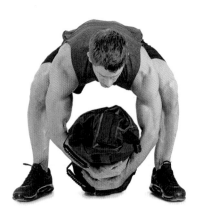

BEAR HUG SQUAT

TARGET MUSCLES: calves, chest, core, glutes, hamstrings, quadriceps, and shoulders

SETUP: Stand tall with your feet slightly wider than shoulder-width apart and toes pointing out at an angle. Position a sandbag vertically (with one end facing you) on the floor between your feet. Bear hug the sandbag up to your chest.

PUSH: Keeping your head and back straight, push your hips back and slowly squat down until your thighs are parallel to the floor. (Your knees should be directly above your toes; avoid letting them extend past your feet.) Push yourself back up into a standing position, knees unlocked, and repeat.

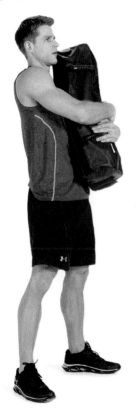
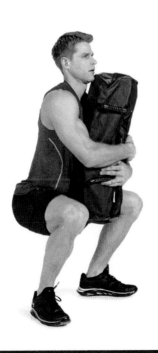

PERFORMANCE POINTERS

CHOOSE THE RIGHT WEIGHT. Selecting a sandbag that's too heavy to hold may tire out your arms before your legs get a thorough workout. Instead of going too heavy, pick a sandbag that you are able to manage without having to quit too soon.

TAKE LONGER TO GET UP. Pause for more than 1 second at the bottom—try 2 or 3, for a real burn—and your quadriceps, hamstrings, and glutes will stay contracted for a longer period of time.

OPTION

WIDE-STANCE BEAR HUG SQUAT

Space your feet about twice as wide as shoulder-width apart and perform the exercise as explained.

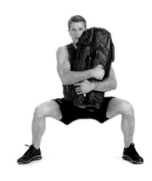

CLEAN

To get into the starting position for many sandbag exercises, you will be asked to "clean the bag," which has nothing to do with soap and water. This is both a positioning move and its own exercise.

TARGET MUSCLES: back, chest, core, glutes, and legs

SETUP: Stand with your feet shoulder-width apart and a sandbag lying on the floor horizontally in front of your feet. Push your hips back, bend your knees slightly, and reach down to grab the sandbag with both hands.

IF YOUR SANDBAG HAS HANDLES: Grab the handles with your palms facing in.

IF YOU DON'T HAVE HANDLES ON A MEDIUM-SIZE SANDBAG: Grab each end of the bag with a neutral grip, palms facing in.

IF YOU DON'T HAVE HANDLES ON A LARGE SANDBAG: Grab the top of the sandbag with an overhand grip, hands shoulder-width apart.

Your arms should hang straight down in front of you, shoulders pulled back, with your weight resting on your heels.

PULL: In one move, explosively pull the sandbag upward toward your shoulders by pushing your hips forward and driving your feet into the floor to straighten your legs.

As the sandbag comes above your waist, you have several options, depending on which exercise you are preparing to do.

TO PERFORM A BASIC CLEAN OR TO GET IN POSITION TO DO A SQUAT, LUNGES, OR ANY EXERCISE THAT REQUIRES HOLDING THE BAG AT CHEST LEVEL: Rotate your forearms under the sandbag to allow it to roll up and into the crooks of your arms, close to your chest. Or, if you don't have handles, you can quickly bring your arms underneath the bag to catch it in the crooks of your arms.

FOR PRESSING EXERCISES: Rotate your forearms under the sandbag to allow it to roll up and over your knuckles, catching it so that the sandbag is above your hands at shoulder height, elbows pointing down.

You should end up in a standing position, back straight and elbows down, with the sandbag in front of your shoulders. Reverse the motion by flipping the sandbag over, unhinging your hips, and bending your knees slightly to lower the sandbag back into the Setup position. Or, if possible, you can also choose to drop the sandbag in front of your feet.

PERFORMANCE POINTERS

HAVE WIGGLE ROOM.
Keep your feet flat at the start, but be sure you can wiggle your toes. That will tell you that the weight is loaded more along the back of your body.

DIP DOWN TO CATCH.
Quickly dropping into a slight squat at the top of the movement can help you get under the sandbag to catch it, which brings your lower body more into the movement.

KEEP YOUR ARMS IN CLOSE.
The farther you extend them away from your body when lifting and lowering the sandbag, the harder the sandbag will bang into your arms and upper body at the top—or pull you forward upon returning it to the floor.

WATCH YOUR POSTURE.
Keep the sandbag close to your body and always brace your core as if you are expecting a punch in the gut.

KEEP ELBOWS DOWN.
If your elbows are up in front of you, your shoulders and arms are doing more work to keep the bag in place than your back and legs are.

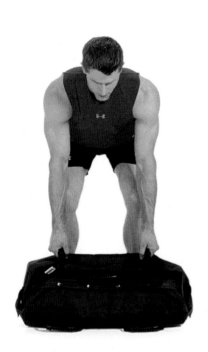

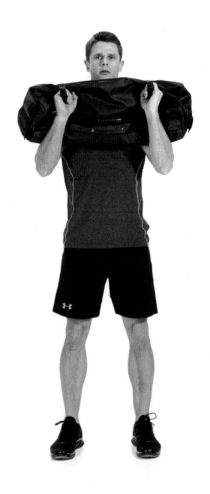

SHOULDERING

Many unilateral movements, where you load the weight on one side of your body, will require you to drape the sandbag over one shoulder in the starting position. Like a clean, shouldering a sandbag—lifting it from the floor to your shoulder in one explosive movement—requires a coordinated effort from your core, upper body, and legs that also challenges your balance.

TARGET MUSCLES: total body (biceps, calves, core, forearms, hamstrings, hips, pectorals, quadriceps, shoulders, and upper and lower back)

SETUP: Stand tall with your feet slightly wider than shoulder-width apart and toes pointing out at an angle. Position a sandbag vertically (with one end facing you) on the floor between your feet.

PULL: Keeping your back arched, push your hips back, bend your knees, and squat down, cupping your fingers around both sides of the middle of the sandbag. Lift the sandbag off the floor and up to your shoulder by quickly pushing your hips forward, extending your knees, and squeezing your glutes. Simultaneously pull the sandbag close to your body and place it over your shoulder. The middle of the sandbag should rest on your shoulder to distribute its weight evenly, with your hands still holding the sandbag.

To lower the sandbag, quickly reverse the motion by drawing the sandbag off your shoulder while pushing your hips back and bending your knees. As you squat down, keep the sandbag close to your body and place it back on the floor.

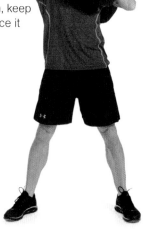

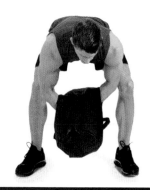

INTERTWINE YOUR HANDS.
Lacing your fingers together underneath the bag will give you more support as you pull.

USE MOMENTUM.
Don't try to muscle the bag up using your arms. Your hips should provide enough power as you rise to help pull the sandbag off the floor and toward your shoulder. Your arms should only be used to position the sandbag over your shoulder at the top of the movement.

STAY ON YOUR HEELS.
You should be able to wiggle your toes before you pull the sandbag from the floor.

GRAB THE SIDES OF THE BAG.
This alternative helps to strengthen your grip and forearms by making your hands work harder throughout the movement. Grasp the sides of the bag with your fingers rather than cupping your hands underneath.

OPTIONS

ONE-ARM SHOULDERING

Take a deep squat, thread your right arm underneath the middle of the bag, and grab it on the opposite side (where your other hand would be). The bag should be resting on the inside of your forearm, and your left arm should hang at your side. Perform the required number of repetitions as explained on the opposite page, switch sides, and repeat.

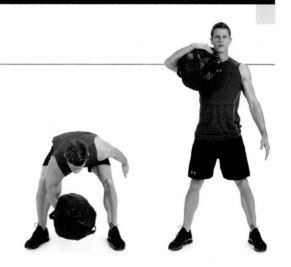

SIDE LUNGE SHOULDERING

Starting with the sandbag shouldered on your left shoulder, step out to your right side into a Side Lunge, and touch the sandbag to the floor. (Don't return the sandbag to the floor—it should either touch the floor or come as close as possible.) As you push yourself back into a standing position, shoulder the sandbag over your left shoulder once more. Repeat for the required number of reps, switch sides, and repeat the exercise with the sandbag resting on your right shoulder while stepping out to your left side.

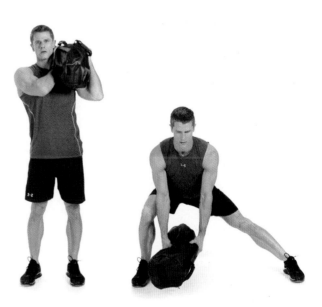

SNATCH

TARGET MUSCLES: total body

SETUP: Stand with your feet shoulder-width apart and a sandbag lying on the floor horizontally (with one long side facing you) in front of your feet. Push your hips back, bend your knees slightly, and reach down to grab the sandbag with both hands—by its handles or with a tight grip at the top, with your hands spaced shoulder-width apart. Your arms should hang straight down in front of you, shoulders pulled back, and your weight should be resting on your heels.

PULL: In one continuous—and explosive—motion, drive your heels into the floor and straighten your legs by driving your hips forward. Simultaneously raise your elbows as high as possible to pull the sandbag upward—imagine you're trying to thrust the sandbag straight up toward the ceiling without letting go of it.

As the sandbag comes above waist height, flip the bag onto your forearms and press it overhead. The sandbag should rotate over your hands—at the top, you should be in a standing position with the sandbag directly above your head, arms straight and locked, palms facing forward.

Reverse the motion to bring the sandbag back into the Setup position, and repeat.

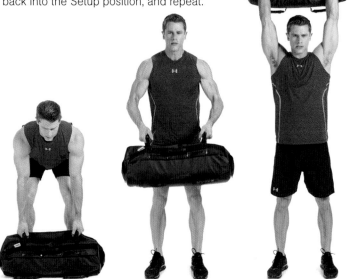

PERFORMANCE POINTERS

STAY VERTICAL.
Keep the sandbag as close to your body as possible at all times.

FOCUS ON THE TOP.
Your arms should line up just behind your ears.

OPTION

ROTATING SNATCH

Get in the Setup position for the Rotating Hang Pull (page 154), but switch to a lighter weight. Perform a snatching motion as you rotate the sandbag over your head and finish at the top in a standing position with the sandbag directly above your head, arms straight and locked, palms facing forward. Return the sandbag to the floor on the opposite side, and repeat.
Extra credit: Includes a Swing!

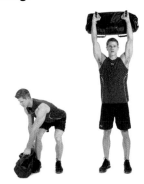

ZERCHER SQUAT

TARGET MUSCLES: biceps, core, legs (primarily the quadriceps), and shoulders

SETUP: Stand with your feet shoulder-width apart and a sandbag lying on the floor horizontally (with one long side facing you) in front of your feet. Clean the sandbag so that it is resting in the crooks of your arms and is pulled in as close to your body as possible.

PUSH: Keeping your torso straight, slowly push your hips back, bend your knees, and squat down until your thighs are parallel to the floor. Push yourself back up until your legs are straight but not locked, and repeat.

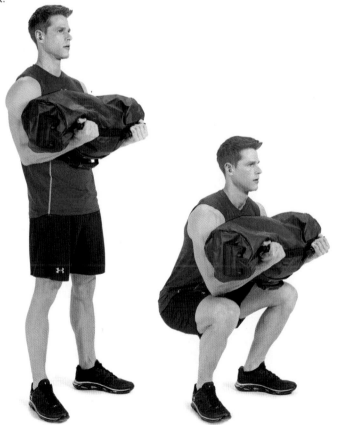

PERFORMANCE POINTERS

WATCH YOUR TOES.
If you feel that your weight is being distributed to the fronts of your feet, you're letting the weight pull you forward. Instead, try to sit back more and push through your heels as you squat.

KEEP ELBOWS DOWN.
If your forearms are too low, your arms will tire out holding the sandbag in position before your legs get a thorough workout.

OPTION

ZERCHER SQUAT AND PRESS

Perform the exercise as explained, but after each squat, press the sandbag overhead and then lower it into the crooks of your arms.

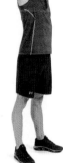

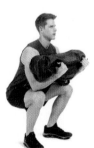

LONG-ARM CRUNCH

TARGET MUSCLE: rectus abdominis

SETUP: Lie flat on your back on a mat or carpeted surface with your knees bent and feet flat. Use both hands to grab a small- to medium-size sandbag and extend your arms over your chest.

PULL: Keeping the sandbag above your torso, slowly pull your head and shoulders 4 to 6 inches off the floor and toward your knees. Pause as you contract your core muscles, lower yourself back down, and repeat.

PERFORMANCE POINTERS

DON'T ROUND YOUR BACK. Instead of rolling up, concentrate on folding your upper body forward, keeping your shoulders and upper back straight as you crunch.

KEEP YOUR FEET FREE. Whenever you anchor your feet during abdominal exercises, you take stress away from your abs and transfer more of the effort onto your hip flexors, the muscles that attach the front of your torso to your legs.

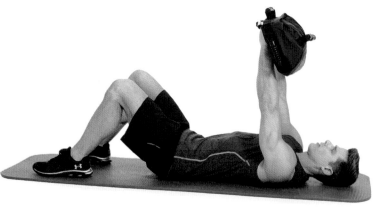

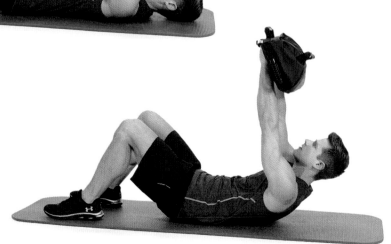

OPTIONS

STANDARD CRUNCH

Wrap your arms around the sandbag as if you've just cleaned it to your shoulders, then keep it on your chest as you lift up off the floor.

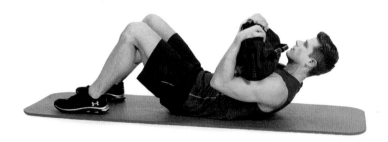

OVERHEAD RAISE
LONG-ARM CRUNCH

Start by lying on your back with your arms behind your head, holding the sandbag. As you crunch up, slowly swing your arms—and the bag—over your head. Stop when the sandbag reaches your knees, then reverse the movement to lower yourself back down.

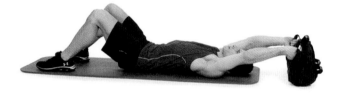

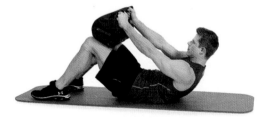

ROTATING CLEAN

TARGET MUSCLES: back, chest, core, glutes, hamstrings, and quadriceps

SETUP: Stand with your feet shoulder-width apart and a sandbag lying on the floor horizontally (with one long side facing you) in front of your feet. Clean the sandbag to the front of your shoulders.

PULL AND SWING: Twist at your waist, swing your torso to the left, let the sandbag rotate over your forearms, and lower it down to the outside of your left leg. At the same time, push your hips back, bending your knees slightly, and allow your right heel to come off the floor as you pivot off the ball of your right foot.

Reverse direction and return to the Setup position by pulling the sandbag upward and cleaning it to your shoulders as you push your hips forward and drive your feet into the floor to straighten your legs. (You should end up in a standing position, back straight and elbows down, with the sandbag in front of your shoulders.) Perform the required number of repetitions, switch sides, and repeat the exercise, this time twisting to your right and lowering the sandbag to your right side.

MASTER THE CLEAN FIRST. Make it your goal to be able to do the clean perfectly before adding any rotating movement to the exercise.

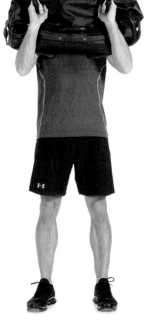
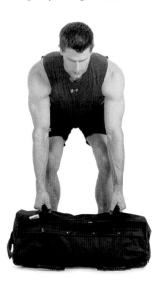
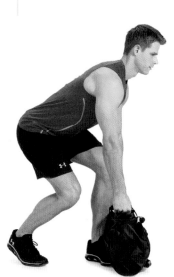

OPTIONS

ROTATING CLEAN AND PRESS

After every clean—every time you're back in the Setup position—immediately press the sandbag overhead, then lower it before the next repetition.

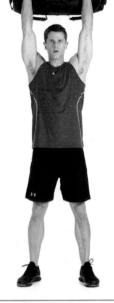
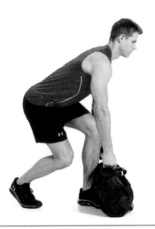
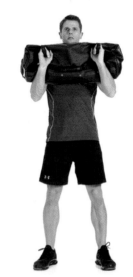

ROTATING CLEAN LUNGE PRESS

After every clean—every time you're back in the Setup position—immediately take a big step forward with either leg and lunge down until your front thigh is parallel to the floor. Push the sandbag over your head, lower it back down to your shoulders, then push yourself back up into the Setup position. Alternate which leg you step forward.

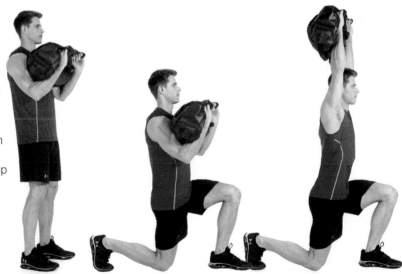

ROTATING DEADLIFT

TARGET MUSCLES: glutes, hamstrings, lower back, quadriceps, trapezius, calves, and core

SETUP: Stand with your feet shoulder-width apart and a sandbag lying on the floor horizontally (with one long side facing you) in front of your feet. Reach down and grab the sandbag with both hands—by its handles or with a tight grip at the top, with your hands spaced shoulder-width apart—then stand back up. Your arms should be hanging straight down in front of you, shoulders pulled back, and your weight should be resting on your heels.

PULL AND SWING: Twist at your waist and swing your torso to the right as you simultaneously push your hips back and squat down, placing the sandbag down on the floor alongside your right foot—but don't let go of the bag. Your left heel should rise off the floor as you pivot off the ball of your left foot.

Pause, then reverse the exercise by pushing your hips forward, driving your feet into the floor to straighten your legs and swinging your torso back to center. Push your hips back and squat down once again, this time swinging to the left and placing the sandbag alongside your left foot. That's 1 repetition.

PERFORMANCE POINTERS

KEEP YOUR ARMS STRAIGHT. Resist the urge to raise your shoulders or bend your elbows as you go. The sandbag should stay close to your body as you lift until your legs are straight but not locked.

DON'T ROUND FORWARD. Keeping your shoulders pulled back will prevent you from arching your upper back, which could cause your lower back to bend, as well.

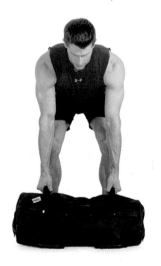
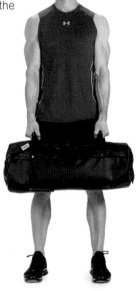
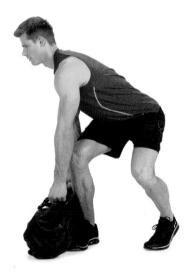

ALTERNATING ROTATING DEADLIFT

Grab the sandbag with the arm farthest from the bag. At the top (when the bag is in front of you), switch the sandbag to the other hand before lowering it back down.

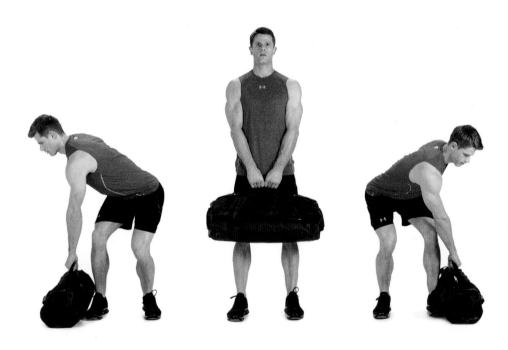

DID YOU KNOW?

You can increase your metabolism by at least 8.5 percent if you eat 18 grams of protein prior to a training session, according to research in the journal *Medicine and Science in Sports and Exercise.*

SHOVELING

TARGET MUSCLES: shoulders, back, and core, especially the obliques, hips, and glutes

SETUP: Stand with feet about shoulder-width apart. Hold a sandbag's parallel handles, with palms facing each other, so the bag rests in front of your thighs as you assume a stable athletic stance.

SWING: Pivot on your left foot to start the bag moving to your right side. You will twist your torso and dip your knees slightly as you lower the bag along your right side (but don't bend over to let it touch the floor). The hip under the bag will project the bag back up as you straighten that right leg and pivot that right foot to swing the bag across your body to the left side. Continue moving the sandbag from side to side. As you twist and pivot from side to side, the motion will feel more like you're swinging a shovel, instead of lifting and lowering the weight.

PERFORMANCE POINTERS

MOVE SLOWLY.
This rotational move teaches how to produce and absorb force under control. Begin with slow swings and concentrate on every segment of the movement.

SPEED UP.
As you become more proficient, move the bag more dynamically from side to side, using your hips and the pivot to generate more power. This gives you a greater metabolic benefit from the exercise.

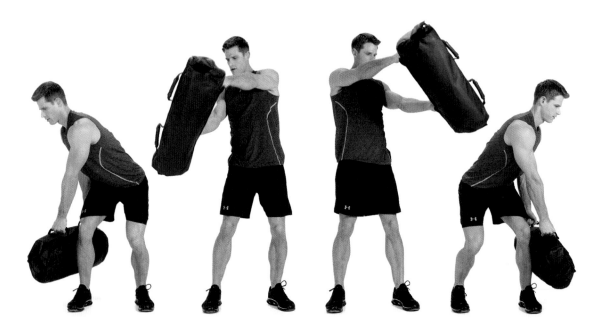

SHUCKING

TARGET MUSCLES: shoulders, low back, hips, and core

SETUP: Take an extra-wide stance with feet wider than shoulder-width apart. Grasp a sandbag by the parallel handles with palms facing each other and let the bag pull your arms straight in front of you between your legs. Now hinge at the hips and remain in this bent-over position.

SWING: Without rising up, swing the sandbag to the right, straightening your left leg and bending your right knee to lower the bag to the floor outside your right foot. Immediately reverse the direction, straightening the right leg and bending the left to swing the bag across your body to the left. Without letting go of the bag, let it touch the floor. Continue shucking the bag back and forth across your body.

PERFORMANCE POINTERS

STAY HINGED.
Fight the urge to stand. Push your hips back as if trying to close a door with your butt and stay in that position throughout the shucking.

SPEED UP.
You can increase the metabolic demands of the exercise by moving the bag faster. You can also make it harder by using a heavier bag.

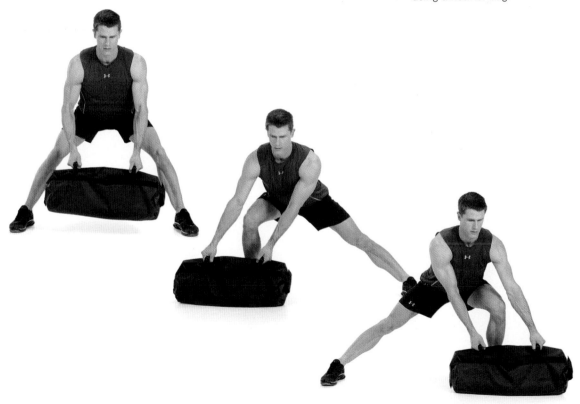

ROTATING HANG PULL

TARGET MUSCLES: biceps, calves, core, glutes, hamstrings, posterior deltoids, quadriceps, and upper and lower back

SETUP: Stand with your feet shoulder-width apart and a sandbag lying on the floor horizontally (with the long side facing you) in front of your feet. Reach down and grab the sandbag with both hands—by its handles or with a tight grip at the top, with your hands spaced shoulder-width apart—then stand back up. Your arms should be hanging straight down in front of you, shoulders pulled back, and your weight should be resting on your heels.

PULL AND SWING: Twisting at your waist, swing your torso to the right and lower the sandbag down by pulling your hips back until your hands are even with your right knee. At the same time, raise your left heel off the floor and pivot on the ball of your left foot.

In one move, pull the sandbag up to shoulder height by drawing your elbows up as you simultaneously squeeze your glutes, push your hips forward, and twist to the left. Bring the sandbag back down to your left side—this time raising your right heel off the floor and pivoting off the ball of your right foot—until your hands are even with your left knee. That's 1 repetition.

PERFORMANCE POINTERS

GET THE TEMPO DOWN. Don't rush the movement—perform it slowly until you get in the rhythm of the exercise.

FACE FORWARD AT THE TOP. By the time you've pulled the sandbag directly up in front of you, both of your feet should be pointing straight ahead (not pivoting) and your elbows should be high.

OPTION

ROTATING HIGH PULL

Perform the exercise as explained, but start with the bag on the floor to increase your range of motion. Place the bag on the floor after each pull.

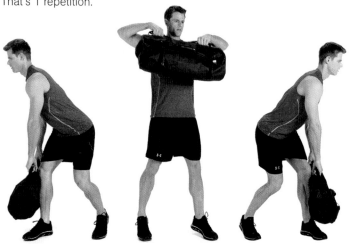

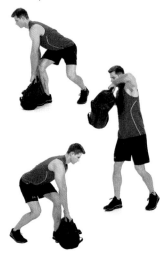

AROUND-THE-WORLD

TARGET MUSCLES: back, core, and shoulders

SETUP: Use a light sandbag for this rotational core exercise. Stand tall with your feet shoulder-width apart. Use both hands to hold a sandbag—by its handles or by gripping the top or sides of the bag—in front of your thighs. Contract your core muscles and keep them braced throughout the exercise because the stress on your trunk changes constantly as you move in opposition to the movement of the bag.

SWING: Slowly swing the sandbag up to your left and behind your head as you swing your torso to the right, raising your right heel off the floor as you pivot on the ball of your right foot. As the sandbag reaches the back of your head, rotate your body back to the center so that you end up facing forward with the bag directly behind your shoulders. Continue the movement by slowly lowering the sandbag to your right side as you swing your torso to the left, raising your left heel off the floor and pivoting on the ball of your left foot. Bring the bag back in front of your thighs in the Setup position. Perform the required number of repetitions, then stop and rotate the bag in the opposite direction for the required number of repetitions.

PERFORMANCE POINTERS

THINK COUNTERINTUITIVELY. Imagine your body moving around the sandbag, not the sandbag going around you. This will help you concentrate on engaging more of your core muscles and performing the move with control.

PICK UP THE TEMPO. Once you've demonstrated that you can do the move slowly and with control, start moving your feet and the bag at a quicker pace.

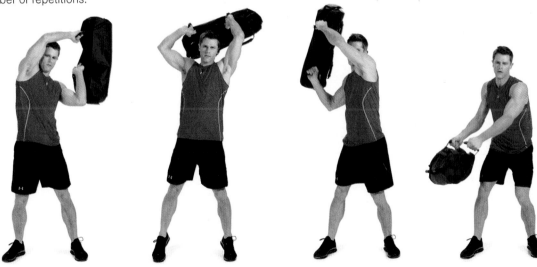

ROTATING LUNGE

TARGET MUSCLES: biceps, calves, core, glutes, hamstrings, posterior deltoids, quadriceps, and upper and lower back

SETUP: Stand with your feet shoulder-width apart and a sandbag lying on the floor horizontally (with one long side facing you) in front of your feet. Reach down and grab the sandbag with both hands—by its handles or with a tight grip at the top, with your hands spaced shoulder-width apart—then stand back up. Your arms should be hanging straight down in front of you, shoulders pulled back, and your weight should be resting on your heels.

PUSH AND SWING: Take a big step backward with your left foot and lower your body until your right thigh is parallel to the floor. Simultaneously twist your waist to the right and swing the sandbag down to the outside of your front (right) leg. Reverse the motion by driving your hips forward and pushing yourself back into the Setup position, then repeat.

Performed the required number of repetitions, switch sides, and repeat.

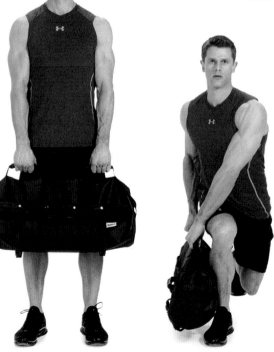

PERFORMANCE POINTERS

KEEP YOUR ARMS STRAIGHT.
Your hips should be doing the bulk of the work. Don't bend your elbows to help keep your arms from helping you swing the weight.

BEGIN SLOWLY.
Do the movement slowly and under control until you master the exercise. Then, gradually increase your speed.

ONE SIDE AT A TIME.
Do this until you feel comfortable with the exercise. Then try alternating sides quickly.

OPTIONS

ALTERNATING ROTATING LUNGE

Perform the exercise as explained on the opposite page, but alternate the movement by stepping back with your left foot (swinging the bag to your right), standing up, and then stepping back with your right foot (swinging the bag to your left).

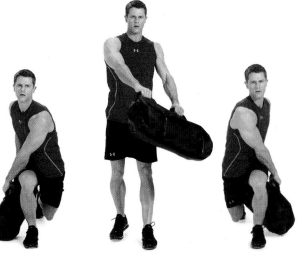

ROTATING LUNGE CLEAN

Begin with the sandbag cleaned to your shoulders. As you step back with one foot, twist and lower the sandbag to the opposite side. Stand back up as you simultaneously clean the sandbag—you should be back in a standing position with the sandbag cleaned to your shoulders—and repeat to the opposite side.

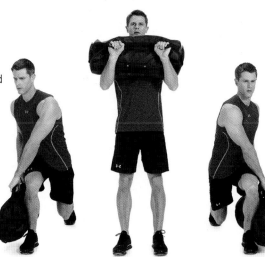

CLEAN AND PRESS

TARGET MUSCLES: back, chest, core, glutes, legs, shoulders, and triceps

SETUP: Stand with your feet shoulder-width apart and a sandbag lying on the floor horizontally in front of your feet.

PUSH AND PULL: Clean the sandbag so that the bag is close to the front of your shoulders, with your knuckles facing up and elbows pointing down. Immediately push your heels into the floor, dip down a few inches by bending your knees, and push the sandbag up over your head. Reverse the motion to lower the sandbag back down to your shoulders, then back down to the floor, and repeat.

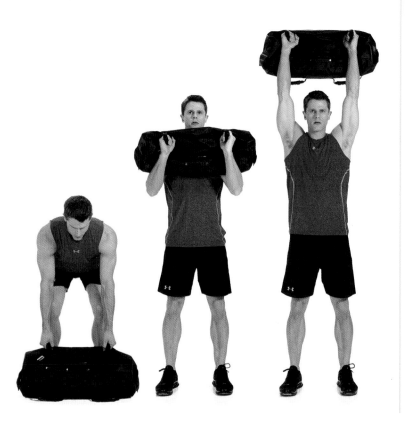

PERFORMANCE POINTERS

HAVE WIGGLE ROOM.
Keep your feet flat at the start, but be sure you can wiggle your toes. That will tell you that the weight is loaded more along the back of your body.

PUSH THROUGH YOUR HEELS.
This will give you more power when pushing the weight directly overhead.

OPTION

STAGGERED STANCE CLEAN AND PRESS

Place one foot behind the other so that the toes of your back foot are in line with the heel of your front foot and your feet are hip-width apart. Perform the exercise as explained, keeping your back heel raised throughout. Perform the required number of repetitions, switch sides, and repeat.

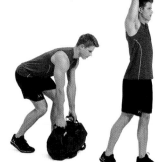

GRIP CURL

TARGET MUSCLES: biceps; also strengthens grip

SETUP: Stand with feet hip-width apart and grasp the center of a sandbag held vertically. Allow your arms to hang straight in front of you.

PUSH: Keeping your back straight, bend your arms to curl the sandbag until your forearms touch your biceps, then lower the sandbag. That's 1 repetition.

PERFORMANCE POINTERS

BRACE YOUR CORE.
To keep your back from bending forward, tighten your abs as if you were expecting to be punched in the gut.

TRY OTHER GRIPS.
Hold the sandbag by the handles in the center or at the sides of the bag or grasp the leather or canvas flaps. Changing your grip works your arms from different angles.

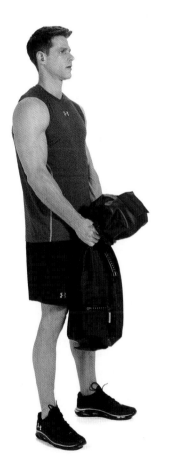 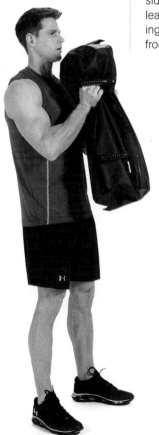

DRAG

TARGET MUSCLES: biceps, calves, core, forearms, glutes, hamstrings, hands, hips, quadriceps, and upper and lower back

SETUP: Thread a rope, 14 to 18 feet long, through the straps of a heavy sandbag, then turn and face away from the sandbag. Place the ends of the rope over your shoulders and grab each end with a fist to keep it in place. Step forward until the rope is taut.

PULL: Starting from a slightly bent-over position (your body should be leaning in front of your feet), quickly run forward, keeping your chest up and back arched as you go. Don't round your back—you should feel the move in your hips, not your spine. Pull the bag behind you for the required amount of time.

PERFORMANCE POINTERS

FOCUS ON YOUR HIPS.
The less they wiggle as you go—you do *not* want to look as if you're using a Hula-Hoop—the better your form will be (and the greater your results).

UTILIZE YOUR SPACE.
If you run out of room as you drag the bag, simply turn around by making a wide circle and travel back the way you came.

DIFFERENT SURFACES, DIFFERENT RESISTANCE.
The weight should be heavy enough that it's hard to pull, but definitely not impossible—but the weight you should use depends on the type of surface you're planning to pull the sandbag on. If it's a rubberized gym floor, placing a towel under the sandbag will help it slide, but you can perform the exercise on grass, sand, and even pavement.

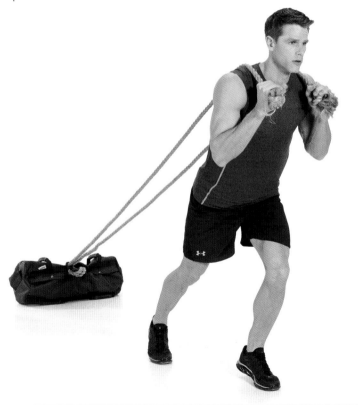

OPTIONS

OFFSET DRAG

Place both ends of the rope over one shoulder so that one side of your body feels more of the effort. Perform the exercise as explained on the opposite page.

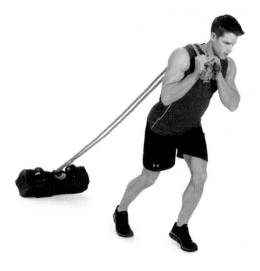

ONE-ARM DRAG

If you don't have a rope, stand to the side of one end of the bag, grab it with one hand, then shuffle away from the bag, dragging it with your arm extended down toward the floor. Repeat with the opposite arm.

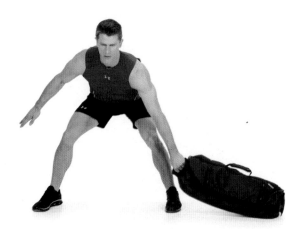

FARMER'S WALK

TARGET MUSCLES: calves, forearms, glutes, grip, hamstrings, quadriceps, and traps

SETUP: Stand with your feet shoulder-width apart and a sandbag lying on the floor horizontally (with one long side facing you) in front of your feet. Clean the sandbag so that the bag is resting in the crooks of your arms, close to your body.

PUSH: Pushing off the balls of your feet, walk forward for the required time or distance.

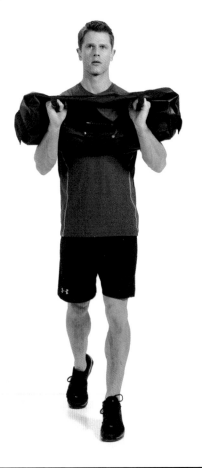

PERFORMANCE POINTERS

UTILIZE YOUR SPACE.
If you don't have enough room to walk, you can either walk in a circle or in a figure-eight pattern, both of which require far less space.

RAISE YOUR HEELS.
Balancing on the balls of your feet will shift extra effort onto your calf muscles.

TRY TO PICK UP THE PACE.
Once you feel comfortable with the exercise, try to increase the tempo of your stride. Using a sandbag (as opposed to dumbbells or kettlebells) makes it easier to sprint without worrying about hitting yourself with the weight.

DID YOU KNOW?

When your resistance-training workouts call for a rest in between exercises or circuits, consider jumping rope for 1 minute. Then rest for 30 seconds to 1 minute before doing your next set. Doing so can nearly double the calories you burn during a workout.

OPTIONS

OFFSET FARMER'S WALK

Shoulder the sandbag on one side, then walk forward for half the required time or distance. Switch the sandbag to your opposite shoulder and finish the exercise.

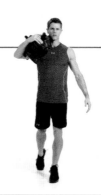

BEAR HUG FARMER'S WALK

Grab the sandbag in a bear hug hold, making sure the bottom end is high enough to allow you to walk comfortably. Perform the exercise as explained on the opposite page.

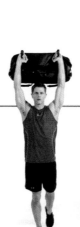

OVERHEAD FARMER'S WALK

Grab a lighter sandbag than you would typically use for the Farmer's Walk, then clean and push it over your head before you perform the exercise.

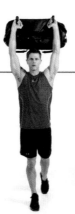

ONE-ARM OVERHEAD FARMER'S WALK

Grab a smaller sandbag with one hand and push it over your head before you walk. Walk forward for half the required time or distance, then switch the weight to your opposite hand and finish the exercise.

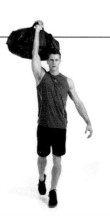

GETUP

TARGET MUSCLES: core, glutes, hamstrings, hips, lower back, and quadriceps

SETUP: Lie flat on your back with a sandbag draped over your left shoulder. Your left arm should be wrapped around the middle of the sandbag, and your right arm should be extended at your side. Bend your left leg and place your left foot flat on the floor, and extend your right leg.

PUSH: Keeping your left arm wrapped around the sandbag, stand up. Begin by rolling onto your right side to help prop yourself up on your right elbow, then push up with your right arm so you're resting on your right hand.

Push yourself up into a half-kneel by threading your right leg behind your left leg. From there, stand up, keeping the sandbag lying vertically over your left shoulder at all times. Reverse the steps to return to the Setup position. Perform the required number of repetitions, switch sides, and repeat.

KEEP YOUR FOOT ON THE FLOOR. Pushing the foot of your bent leg into the floor at all times will help you distribute the load more evenly and allow you to utilize more muscles, including your glutes and hips, for more strength and power.

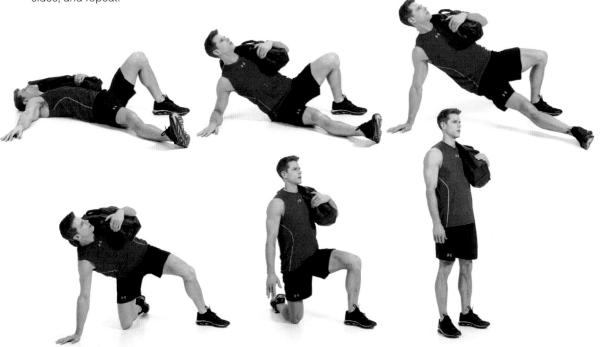

SIDE CRUNCH HIP THRUST

Perform the exercise as explained on the opposite page, but only go as far as rolling onto your side and propping yourself up on your supporting arm, then push your hips up so that your torso forms a straight line with your thighs.

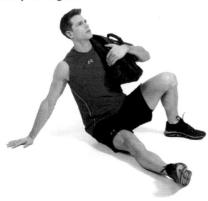
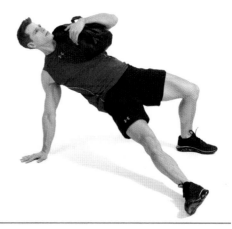

BOTTOM-HALF GETUP
(ALSO CALLED SHOULDER LEG THREADING)

Perform the exercise as explained on the opposite page, but only go as far as rolling onto your side, propping yourself up, and threading your straight leg under the leg that is bent and on the side of the bag. Then return to the Setup position.

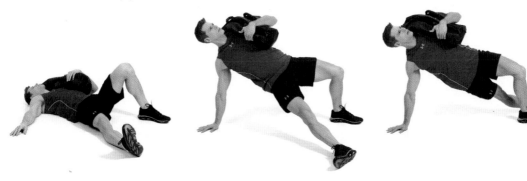

TURKISH GETUP

TARGET MUSCLES: core, glutes, hamstrings, hips, lower back, and quadriceps

SETUP: Lie flat on your back holding a sandbag in your left hand. Your right arm should be extended, palm flat on the floor. Straighten your left arm so that the weight is directly above you and the bag rests on your forearm.

PUSH: Keeping your left elbow locked and the weight above you at all times, stand up in this sequence: Begin by rolling onto your right side, then push up with your right arm so you are resting on your right hand. Thread your right leg behind your left leg and put your knee on the ground. Push your torso upright to get into a half-kneeling stance. Begin to stand up, keeping the bag above you at all times.

Keeping your left arm straight, reverse the steps to return to the Setup position, then repeat. Perform the required number of repetitions, switch sides, and repeat.

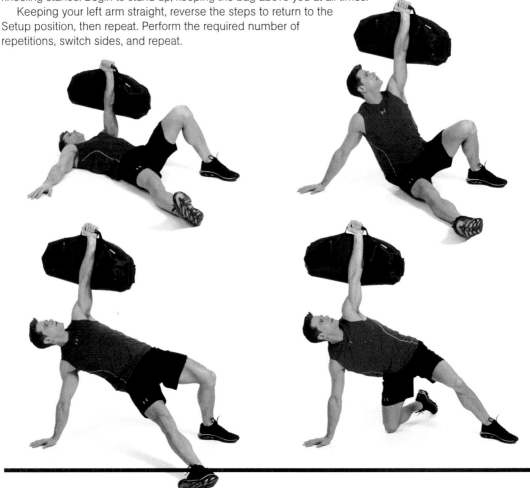

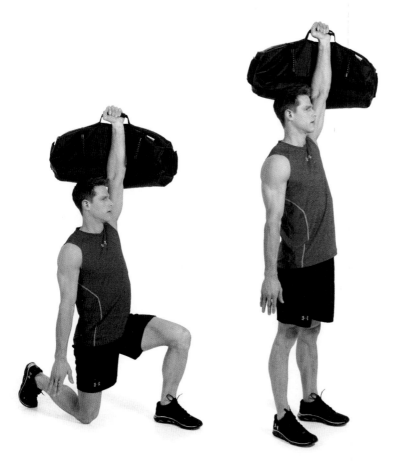

PERFORMANCE POINTERS

KEEP YOUR EYE ON THE BAG.
Imagine that the goal of the entire move is to simply push the weight straight up toward the ceiling.

KEEP YOUR FOOT ON THE FLOOR. Pushing the foot of your bent leg into the floor at all times will help you distribute the load more evenly and allow you to utilize more muscles, including your glutes and hips, which will give you more strength and power.

GOOD MORNING

TARGET MUSCLES: glutes, hamstrings, and lower back

SETUP: Stand with your feet shoulder-width apart and a sandbag lying on the floor horizontally in front of your feet. Clean the sandbag so that the bag is resting in the crooks of your arms.

PULL: With your knees unlocked and your back flat, push your hips back and slowly bend at your waist until your torso is almost parallel to the floor. The sandbag should remain locked close to your chest with your arms wrapped around it. Slowly pull your torso back up into the Setup position, and repeat.

PERFORMANCE POINTER

BRACE YOUR CORE.
Contract your abs, then hold them in that contracted state. (Imagine that you're expecting to be punched in the stomach at any time.)

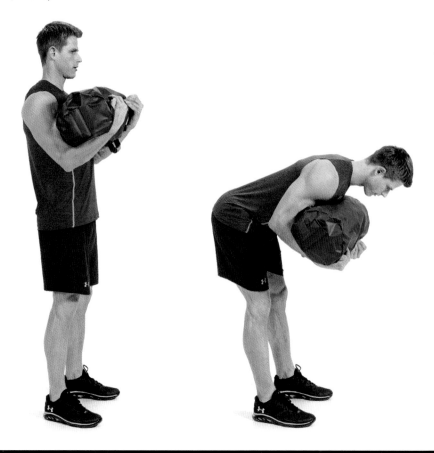

OPTIONS

GOOD MORNING FRONT SQUAT

After performing one Good Morning, keep the sand-bag close to your shoulders, push your hips back, and bend your knees until your thighs are parallel to the floor.

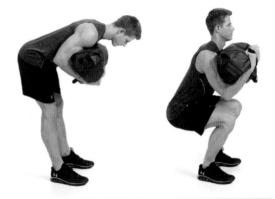

BEAR HUG GOOD MORNING

Bear hug a smaller sandbag that allows you to bend forward at your waist, and perform the exercise as explained on the opposite page.

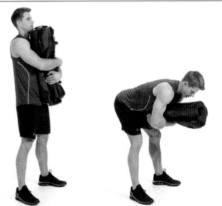

SINGLE-LEG GOOD MORNING

Raise one leg up straight behind you so that when you bend at your waist, your back leg stays in line with your torso. Perform the required number of rep-etitions, switch sides, and repeat.

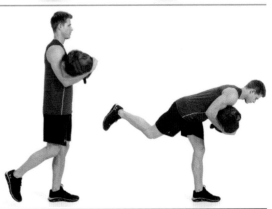

PUSHUP

TARGET MUSCLES: chest, core, shoulders, and triceps

SETUP: Kneel on the floor and get into a pushup position with your arms straight, hands shoulder-width apart, and legs extended behind you. Have a training partner place a sandbag either horizontally across the top of your back and shoulders or, if the sandbag is loose enough, along the length of your torso.

PUSH: Bend your elbows and slowly lower your chest down toward the floor, being careful that the sandbag doesn't shift. Slowly push yourself back up until your arms are straight but not locked, and repeat.

PERFORMANCE POINTER

GO FOR EXTRA REPETITIONS. Once you're reached the point where you're 1 or 2 repetitions away from failure, remove the sandbag and continue to perform pushups.

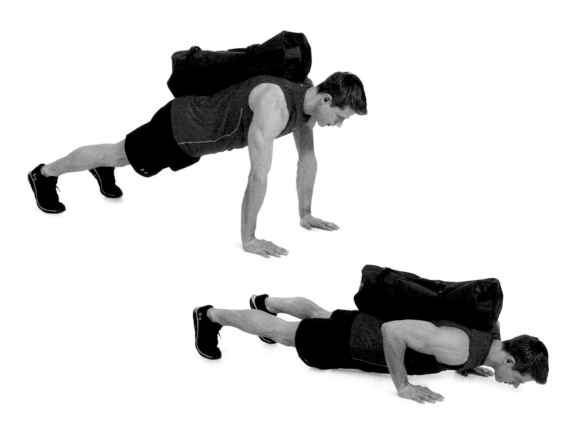

SIDE-TO-SIDE PICKUP

TARGET MUSCLES: lower back, obliques, and rectus abdominis

SETUP: Sit on a mat or carpeted surface with your legs extended in front of you. Place a small- to medium-size sandbag alongside your left hip.

PULL AND SWING: Keeping your legs on the floor and your torso upright, twist your torso to the left, grab the ends of the sandbag with both hands, pick up the sandbag, and rotate your torso to the right to swing the sandbag to your right side. Place the sandbag on the floor alongside your right hip—keeping a grip on the bag the entire time—and reverse the movement, rotating your torso and the bag to your left. That's 1 repetition.

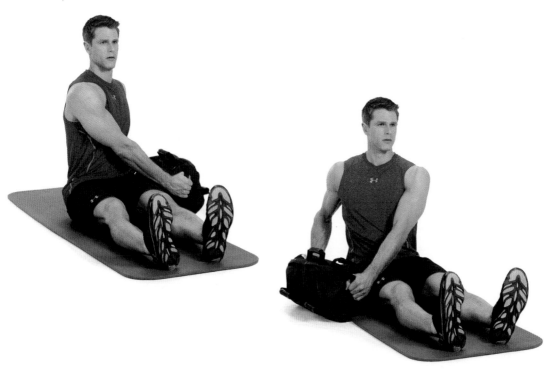

REVERSE LUNGE

TARGET MUSCLES: glutes, hamstrings, quadriceps, and calves

SETUP: Stand with your feet shoulder-width apart and a sandbag lying on the floor vertically (with one end facing you) between your feet. Shoulder the sandbag, placing it over your right shoulder. Wrap your right arm over the end of the sandbag to help keep it in place. Your left arm can hang down at your side.

PUSH: Take a big step backward with your right foot, and lower your body until your left thigh is parallel to the floor. Your right knee should be an inch or two off the floor and should be bent at a 90-degree angle. Only the ball of your right foot should be on the floor.

Quickly reverse the motion by pushing yourself back into the Setup position, and repeat. Perform the required number of repetitions, switch sides, and repeat.

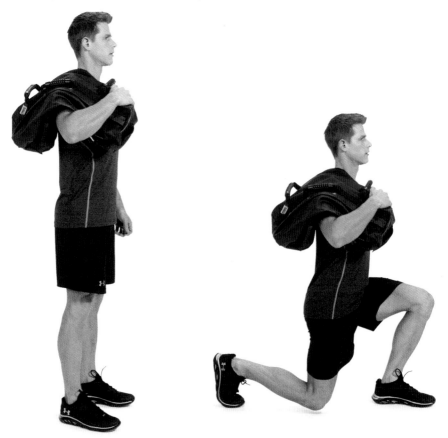

OPTIONS

CLEAN AND LUNGE

Clean the sandbag so that the bag is resting in the crooks of your arms. Step back into a Lunge, push yourself back up, then bring the sandbag to the floor. Clean the sandbag once more, then step back into a Lunge using the opposite leg.

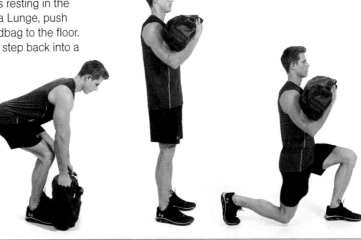

ROTATIONAL REVERSE LUNGE

Hold a sandbag in front of your thighs. Step back with your right foot and swing the bag to the outside of your left thigh. Stand up and return to the starting position. Repeat, switching legs halfway through the set. To increase the difficulty, go into your next Lunge without pausing.

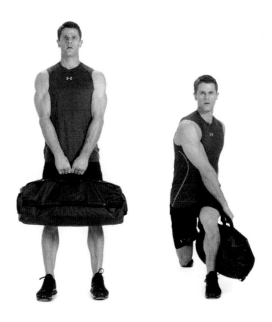

SIDE LUNGE

TARGET MUSCLES: glutes, hamstrings, inner thighs, and quadriceps

SETUP: Stand with your feet shoulder-width apart and a sandbag lying on the floor horizontally in front of your feet. Clean the sandbag so that the bag is resting in the crooks of your arms.

PUSH: Keeping your torso facing forward, take a wide step out to your right with your right foot, and bend your right knee until your right thigh is almost parallel to the floor. Your left leg will be extended and at an angle. Push yourself back up to the Setup position, then take a wide step out to your left with your left foot. Push yourself back to the Setup position. This is 1 rep.

PERFORMANCE POINTERS

STABILIZE YOUR BODY.
Shift your weight onto your heels and keep your core muscles tight to stabilize your spine.

DON'T STEP TOO FAR.
Step far enough that your shin-bone can align itself directly over your placed foot. If it can't, you've gone too far.

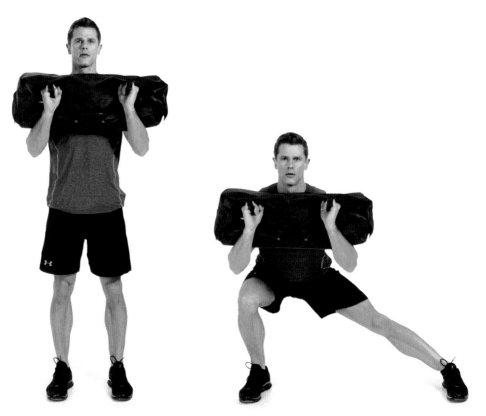

OPTIONS

SIDE LUNGE DEADLIFT

Instead of cleaning the sandbag as explained on the opposite page, let your arms hang straight down in front of you. As you lunge, let the sandbag touch the floor in front of your working foot. ***Extra credit: Includes a Pull!***

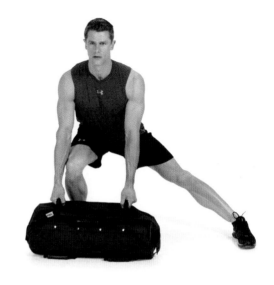

SIDE LUNGE CLEAN

Perform the exercise as explained on the opposite page, but lower the sandbag back down to touch the floor in front of your working foot as you lunge. As you push yourself back up into the Setup position, clean the sandbag back to your shoulders. ***Extra credit: Includes a Pull!***

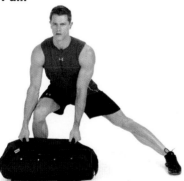
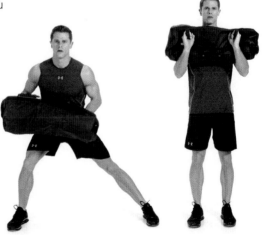

SWING

TARGET MUSCLES: back, core, glutes, and hamstrings

SETUP: Stand with your feet slightly wider than shoulder-width apart and hold a small- to medium-size sandbag with both hands, either from the middle of the bag or from one end. Unlock your knees, push your hips back, and lean forward at your waist. (Your knees will bend slightly as you go.) Your arms should hang straight down in front of you, palms facing back.

PULL: To get the sandbag moving, swing the weight back between your legs. Without rounding your back, quickly push yourself back into a standing position as you squeeze your glutes, thrust your hips forward, and swing the sandbag up and in front of you at about shoulder or head height. Reverse the movement, allowing gravity to bring the sandbag back into the Setup position, and repeat.

PERFORMANCE POINTERS

CHOOSE THE RIGHT SIZE. Unlike dumbbells and kettle-bells, which are more compact in size, the dimensions of a sandbag can make this move challenging if you have shorter legs or a sandbag that's too unwieldy.

DON'T ACTIVELY LIFT. Let the momentum of the exercise swing the bag up to chest or head level and let gravity pull it back down.

OPTION

SINGLE-ARM SWING

Hold a small sandbag at arm's length in front of your waist and perform the exercise as explained. Your nonworking arm can swing along with your working arm. Perform the required number of reps, switch hands, and repeat.

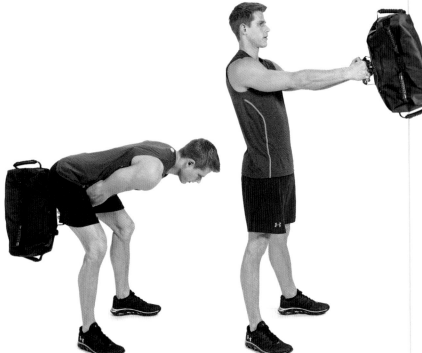

WIPER

TARGET MUSCLE: rectus abdominis

SETUP: On a mat or carpeted surface, lie flat on your back with your knees bent to 90 degrees and feet elevated. Grab a sandbag with both hands and extend your arms above you. (If your sandbag has handles, let the sandbag drape over the backs of your arms.)

SWING: Keeping the sandbag raised above you and your head and back flat on the floor, slowly lower your legs to the right, keeping your feet from touching the floor. Raise your legs to the center and then lower them to the left. That's 1 rep.

PERFORMANCE POINTER

STRAIGHTEN LEGS UPWARD. The farther your feet are from your waist, the harder the exercise will be on your abdominals.

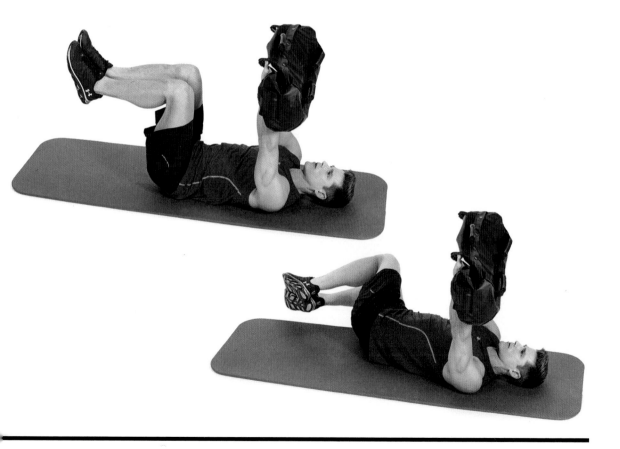

SHOULDER-TO-SHOULDER PRESS

TARGET MUSCLES: core, shoulders, triceps, and upper trapezius

SETUP: Stand tall with your feet slightly wider than shoulder-width apart and toes pointing out at an angle. Position a sandbag vertically on the floor (with one end facing you) between your feet. Shoulder the sandbag up to your right shoulder, keeping a firm grip on the sandbag with both hands.

PUSH: Without using your legs to help you push the bag upward, slowly extend your arms and push the sandbag up and over your head in an arc, and place the sandbag on your left shoulder. Repeat the exercise, moving the sandbag to the opposite shoulder. That's 1 rep.

PERFORMANCE POINTERS

KEEP LEGS STRAIGHT.
The less you bend your knees, the more effort your shoulders, upper back, triceps, and core will make.

RAISE IT UP.
If you have shorter arms, not extending your arms fully when lifting the bag could cause it to hit or scrape your head, which may not hurt you, but it can mess up your tempo.

KEEP YOUR HEAD IN PLACE.
Don't tilt or tip your head to avoid the bag. Your head should remain straight and in line with your back at all times.

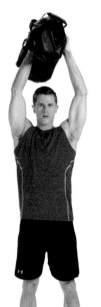

OPTIONS

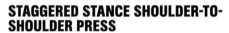

KNEELING SHOULDER-TO-SHOULDER PRESS (ARC PRESS)

Kneel on a mat or carpeted surface with your legs bent at 90 degrees and your toes pressing into the floor. Perform the exercise as explained on the opposite page. This posture puts more emphasis on your core and glutes by removing your legs from the exercise.

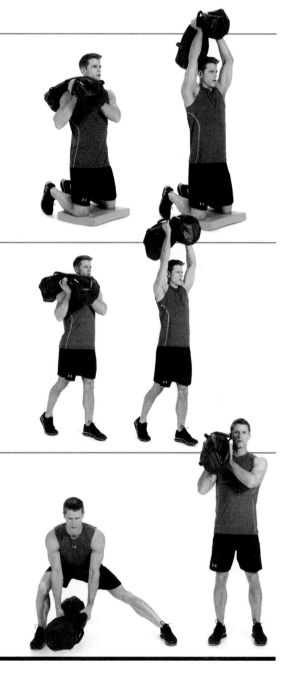

STAGGERED STANCE SHOULDER-TO-SHOULDER PRESS

With feet slightly wider than shoulder-width apart, place one foot back so that the toes of your back foot are in line with the heel of your front foot. Perform the exercise as explained on the opposite page with your back heel raised and only the toes of your back foot on the floor. Perform the required number of repetitions, switch legs, and repeat.

SIDE LUNGE/SHOULDER-TO-SHOULDER PRESS

Perform a Shoulder-to-Shoulder Press from right to left, and then from left to right. Once the sandbag is resting over your right shoulder, step out to the side with your right foot. As you lunge down, lower the sandbag toward the floor, arms extended, but don't let go of the sandbag. Push yourself back into a standing position as you shoulder the sandbag over your right shoulder again, and repeat. Perform the required number of repetitions, switch sides, and repeat.

SINGLE-LEG ROW

TARGET MUSCLES: lats, lower back, middle trapezius, and rhomboids

SETUP: Stand with your feet shoulder-width apart and hold a sandbag horizontally, grabbing it with both hands spaced shoulder-width apart, palms facing in. With your arms hanging down in front of you, raise your right leg behind you, then slowly bend forward at your waist until your back and leg are almost parallel to the floor. Let your arms hang straight down below you.

PULL: Without moving your upper body, pull the sandbag to your chest and squeeze your shoulder blades together. Pause, lower the sandbag, and repeat. After completing reps, switch legs.

PERFORMANCE POINTERS

KEEP A STRAIGHT LINE. Lifting your head or turning your neck may strain your neck muscles. Instead, look down at the floor in front of you as you row.

MOVE ONLY YOUR ARMS. If you find yourself raising your torso or bending and straightening your legs in order to lift the sandbag, you're using more momentum and less muscle.

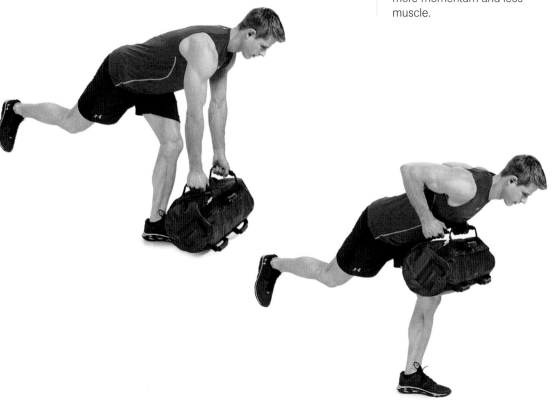

OPTIONS

VERTICAL SINGLE-LEG ROW

Hold the bag vertically, grabbing its sides as if you were going to shoulder it. Perform the exercise as explained on the opposite page.

NEUTRAL-GRIP BENT-OVER ROW

Stand with your feet hip- to shoulder-width apart and position a sandbag horizontally in front of your feet. Hinge at your hips until your torso is parallel to the floor. Grasp the handles or sides of the bag. Keeping a slight bend in your legs but without moving your torso, row the bag to your chest, squeezing your shoulder blades together at the top of the movement. Lower and repeat.

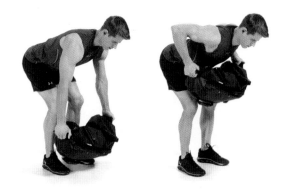

STAGGERED STANCE BENT-OVER ROW

With feet hip-width apart, move one foot back until its toes align with the instep of your other foot. This is the starting position. Perform a Bent-Over Row. Complete all repetitions, then switch foot positions and repeat.

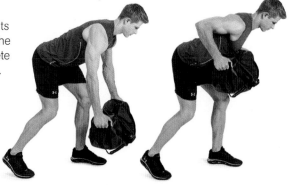

LATERAL DRAG

TARGET MUSCLES: chest, core, latissimus dorsi, shoulders, and triceps

SETUP: Start in a plank position (the top of a pushup) with a small sandbag on the floor next to your left side. Spread your feet slightly wider than shoulder-width apart for greater balance and keep your arms straight and hands flat on the floor directly under your shoulders.

PULL AND SWING: Shift your weight onto your left arm as you reach your right arm underneath your body and grab the sandbag. Drag the bag underneath you until it rests on your right side. Let go of the bag and place your right hand back on the floor to get back into the Setup position. Repeat, this time reaching under with your left hand and dragging the weight to your left side while shifting your weight onto your right arm.

PERFORMANCE POINTERS

MINIMIZE HIP MOVEMENT.
The effort shouldn't come from you twisting at your hips. Instead, keep yourself grounded by pushing through your toes and letting your arms move the weight.

BRING FEET TOGETHER.
The farther apart they are, the easier it is to stay balanced, so spacing them closer together makes the move more challenging.

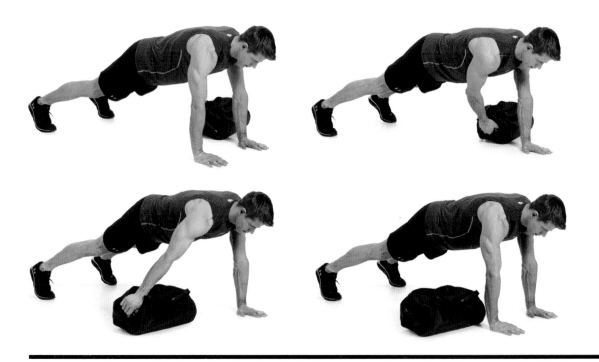

Other Sandbag Exercises to Try

You can substitute a sandbag for a dumbbell (or two sandbags for a pair of dumbbells) in the following exercises shown in the dumbbell chapter.

- Biceps Curl (page 46)
- Chest Press (page 48)
- Crunch (page 51)
- Front Squat (page 53)
- Deadlift (page 56)
- Romanian Deadlift (page 58)
- Straight-Leg Deadlift (page 59)
- Single-Leg Standing Calf Raise (page 63)
- Push Press (page 68)

- Shrug (page 69)
- Kneeling Twist, Russian Twist (page 71)
- Stepup (page 74)
- Two-Arm Row (page 76)
- Single-Leg Woodchop (page 79)
- Reverse Woodchop (page 79)
- Lying Triceps Extension (page 80)
- Overhead Triceps Extension (page 82)
- Standing Shoulder Press (page 84)

You can substitute a sandbag for a kettlebell (or kettlebells) in the following exercises shown in the kettlebell chapter:

- 45-Degree Two-Arm Row (page 99)
- Bent Press (page 101)
- High Pull (page 112)

- Sots Press (page 121)
- Windmill (page 134)

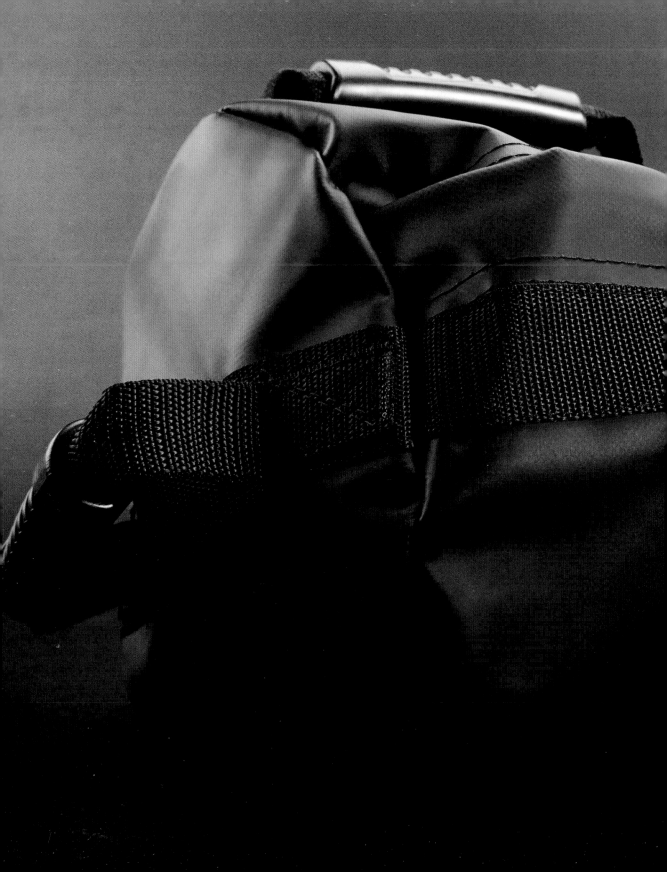

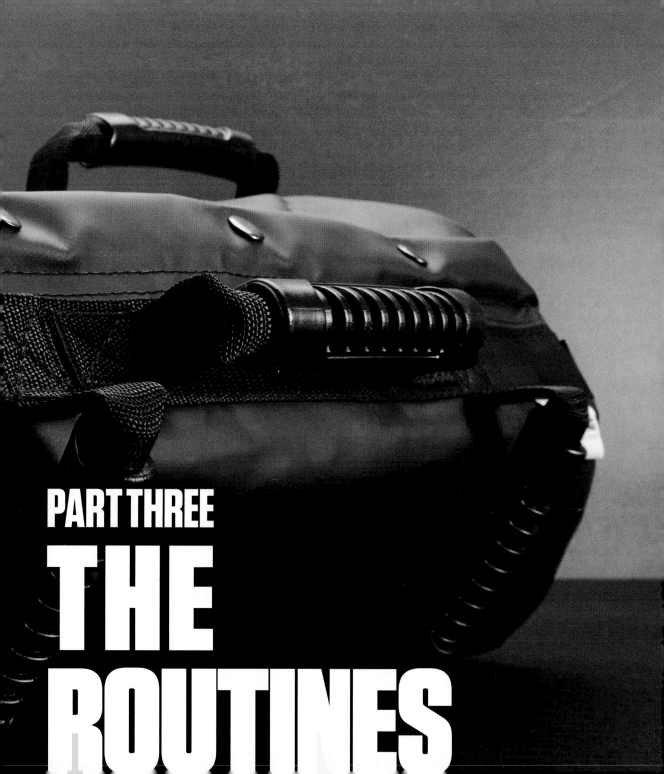

PART THREE
THE ROUTINES

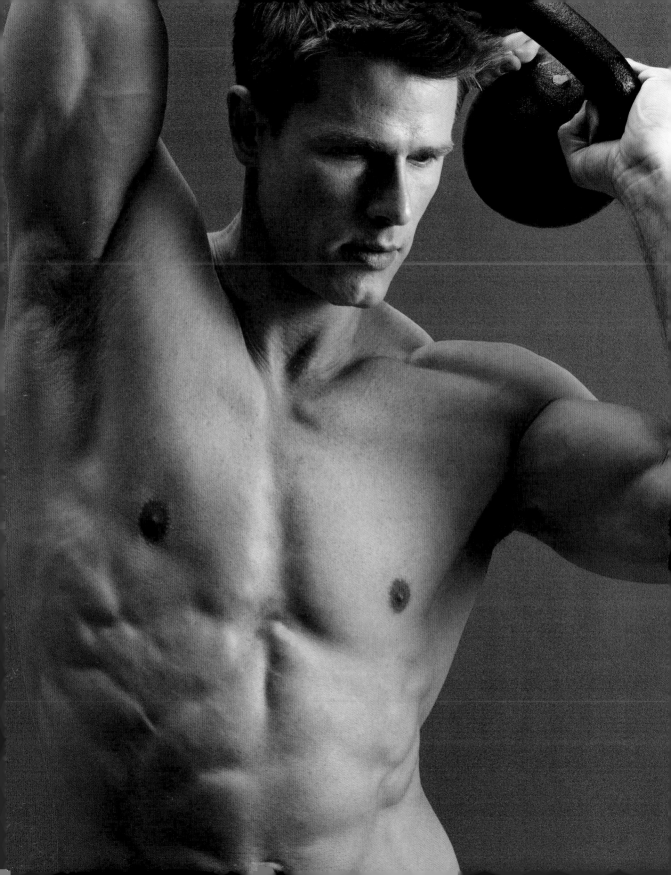

CHAPTER 9

THE TEST DRIVE

1-WEEK TRYOUTS TO LEARN THE KEY MOVES AND SAMPLE EACH PIECE OF GEAR

If you're new to weight training or are not familiar with dumbbells, kettlebells, or sandbags, this is the place to start. It's a beginner's chapter designed to help you familiarize yourself with the equipment and nail some basic moves. For that matter, even if you're an experienced lifter with over a year's worth of training under your belt, take the time to "test drive." Pushing, pulling, and swinging the three pieces of equipment using a short, 1-week routine for each will amplify your performance by helping you perfect your form.

In fact, most experts agree that experienced lifters can take major steps forward in their workouts by downshifting their routines every so often. By returning to the basics, you may find yourself focusing more on the movements you may be taking for granted when pulling off more complex routines. Through downshifting, you may find yourself working out the kinks and mistakes you may have been making on these basic moves, which means that your body—and every muscle challenged during each exercise—will experience a more thorough, muscle-altering workout.

The 1-Week Dumbbell Test Drive

Beginners and even intermediate-level exercisers (those who have been lifting for 6 months to a year) can make the mistake of following advanced programs that involve exercises that are too complex, too muscle-specific, or too redundant. Whether you're fresh to weight lifting, coming back from a long time away, or just ready to be reminded of why the basics are so important, this starting routine is for everyone. No matter what your goal is—size and strength, muscular definition, or fat loss—you can benefit from the "big four" exercises: the Squat, the Chest Press, the Deadlift, and the Two-Arm Row.

These four moves do more than just work every major muscle group—and most of the minor ones—in your body. They also allow you to handle significantly heavier weight loads relative to your strength, which gives your body the greatest potential to release anabolic hormones and stimulate more lean muscle growth. All that extra muscle will not only leave you stronger, it will also help raise your metabolism, turning your body into an all-day fat-burning furnace.

In addition, focusing primarily on these four moves—performed correctly—enables your body to develop a functional foundation that improves your posture, builds core strength, and gives you a better sense of body awareness. This 1-2-3 punch can instantly improve your ability to perform and generate results from many other exercises in this book.

To master these four moves and expose your muscles to multiple variables that change the moves' effect on your body, you need repetition. That's why you'll perform them three times a week, but you'll change certain variables, such as the number of reps and the length of your rest periods between sets. (Typically, you would only use these multijoint, compound exercises once or twice a week, but because this routine is about understanding the movements, your best bet is to temporarily perform them more frequently.)

To bring the swing to the mix, you'll also be performing a fifth move, the Woodchop. This key core stabilization exercise will prepare your midsection and lower back for the workouts you'll be planning and performing once you've built your fitness base.

EXERCISE	DAY 1 SETS/REPS/REST	DAY 2 SETS/REPS/REST	DAY 3 SETS/REPS/REST
Squat (page 54)	3/8/2 minutes	3/10/90 seconds	3/12/1 minute
Chest Press (page 48)	3/8/2 minutes	3/10/90 seconds	3/12/1 minute
Deadlift (page 56)	3/8/2 minutes	3/10/90 seconds	3/12/1 minute
Two-Arm Row (page 76)	3/8/2 minutes	3/10/90 seconds	3/12/1 minute
Woodchop (page 78)	2/15 each side/1 minute	2/15 each side/1 minute	2/15 each side/1 minute

The Routine

This routine is only done 3 days a week because you'll need at least 48 hours between workouts to recover. Giving your muscles enough time to recover between workouts is crucial, so never try to do two workouts back-to-back. Complete all sets of an exercise before moving on to the next exercise in the chart. Stick with the program for at least 1 week, but feel free to use it for an additional 3 to 4 weeks, depending on how comfortable you become with the movements.

The 1-Week Kettlebell Test Drive

There are certain kettlebell exercises that are the staple moves of any routine you'll see. The Swing (see pages 106 and 108) and Clean (see page 90) are two of the most important movements to lock down before you unleash your muscles on the exercises in this book.

This test drive uses the circuit training method: You'll perform 1 set of each exercise, then immediately move on to the next exercise, keeping the amount of time you rest between exercises to a maximum of 30 seconds. After you've completed all five exercises, rest for 2 minutes, then complete the five-move circuit once more.

The Routine

This routine is done 3 days a week, so space out your workouts to give your body at least 48 hours between workouts to recover. Use the program for at least 1 week, but you can continue using it for an additional 3 to 4 weeks in order to perfect certain moves, particularly the Clean and Press and the Swing.

If you do decide to use the routine for an additional few weeks, stick with the sets and reps recommended on Day 3, and try to minimize the amount of time you rest between exercises and circuits. Eventually, your goal should be to move through all five exercises with no rest in between, perform the five-move round four or five times, and only rest for 30 to 60 seconds between each circuit. But for starters, rest for 30 to 60 seconds between sets and 2 minutes between circuits.

EXERCISE	DAY 1 SETS/REPS	DAY 2 SETS/REPS	DAY 3 SETS/REPS
Clean and Press (page 92)	1/6 each arm	1/8 each arm	1/10 each arm
Bent-Over Row (page 98)	1/6 each arm	1/8 each arm	1/10 each arm
Goblet Squat (page 126)	1/6	1/8	1/10
Single-Arm Swing (page 106)	1/6 each arm	1/8 each arm	1/10 each arm
Around-the-Body Pass (page 94)	1/10 each direction	1/15 each direction	1/20 each direction

The 1-Week Sandbag Test Drive

This starter sandbag routine is made up of five exercises designed to familiarize your muscles with certain techniques, lifts, and movements that will help you progress toward intermediate and advanced exercises later on. You'll perform this test drive using the circuit training method: Complete 1 set of each exercise, then immediately move on to the next exercise, keeping the amount of time you rest between exercises to a maximum of 30 seconds. After you've completed all five exercises, rest for 2 minutes, then complete the five-move circuit once more.

The Routine

This 3-day-a-week routine will require you to rest and recover for at least 48 hours between workouts. Use the program for at least 1 week, but you can continue to use it for another 3 to 4 weeks.

If you do continue the routine for an additional few weeks to become more at ease with the motions, stick with the recommended sets and reps from Day 3, and try to minimize the amount of time you rest between exercises and

KNOW THE LINGO

- **REPETITION (OR REP):** A single complete movement of an exercise, from start to finish.
- **SET:** A group of repetitions performed in succession until completion. For example, doing 1 set of 8 repetitions means that you'll need to perform the exercise eight times to complete a single set.
- **CIRCUIT TRAINING:** A style of exercising in which you perform a series of more than three exercises, moving from one exercise to the next with minimal (if any) rest in between.
- **REST INTERVAL (OR REST):** The amount of time you'll wait between sets. How many seconds or minutes you'll be required to wait will depend on the intensity of the exercise, which will depend on how much weight you're lifting and how fast you're lifting it.

circuits. Eventually, your goal should be to move through all five exercises with no rest in between, perform the five-move circuit three or four times, and only rest for 30 to 60 seconds between each circuit.

EXERCISE	DAY 1 SETS/REPS	DAY 2 SETS/REPS	DAY 3 SETS/REPS
Shouldering (page 142)	1/6 each shoulder	1/8 each shoulder	1/10 each shoulder
Rotating Clean (page 148)	5 each side	6 each side	8 each side
Around-the-World (page 155)	1/10 seconds each direction	1/20 seconds each direction	1/30 seconds each direction
Clean and Press (page 158)	1/8	1/10	1/12
Rotating Lunge (page 156)	1/6 each leg	1/8 each leg	1/10 each leg

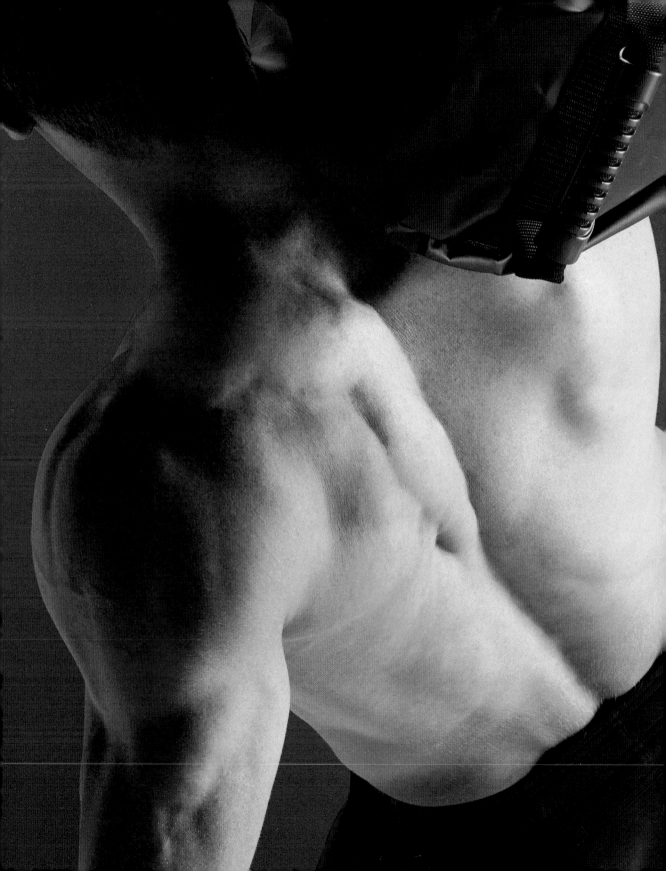

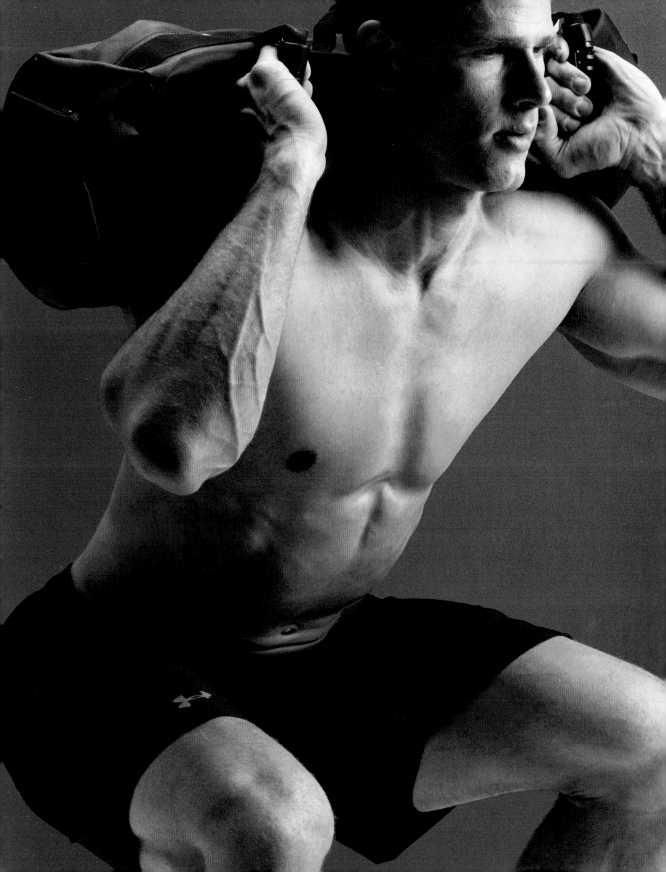

10

BUILD YOUR OWN PUSH, PULL, SWING PROGRAM

CHOOSE A BLEND OF MOVEMENTS FOR TOTAL-BODY FITNESS AND OPTIMUM FAT BURNING

Now that you're primed and ready, it's time to take your workout routines to the next, more challenging level.

Push, Pull, Swing is ultimately a collection of more than 100 great dumbbell, kettlebell, and sandbag exercises—all in one convenient place. If you already know a fair amount about exercise, you can take the moves from the last few chapters and integrate them into your own routines as a way to mix things up,

try something new, and make your workouts less boring—for your mind *and* your muscles. If you simply want to follow a pretested plan or you have a specific goal in mind, you can jump to the next chapter to find all sorts of workout programs for dumbbells, kettlebells, and sandbags. If you want to try building your own workout from the vault of exercises in this book, you're in the right spot. In this chapter, you'll find templates for different

WARM UP OR DON'T LIFT!

Before each and every workout in this chapter and this book, you need to warm up your muscles.

Doing some type of 5-minute, low-intensity activity prior to each workout will help increase bloodflow to your working muscles and increase the elasticity of connective tissues, allowing your muscles to contract more fluidly. Not only will you minimize your risk of injury and improve your performance while exercising, but you'll also recover from your workouts much faster—especially if you perform the same low-intensity activity at the end of each workout as a cooldown.

A few smart, equipment-free choices: Try jogging in place, skipping rope (even without a rope is fine), or jumping jacks.

general workout programs that you can use to achieve your goals. Simply plug the Push, Pull, or Swing exercise you want to do in the appropriate spot in the charts, and you'll automatically ensure that you're getting a solid metabolic workout that attacks your body from all angles.

There are many different ways you can integrate the Push, Pull, Swing method into a workout, depending on what type of routine works best for you. Just remember this simple rule for building routines: The workouts in each week should always incorporate a blend of upper body push and pull exercises, lower body push and pull exercises, and swing or core movements.

If you take a look at all three 1-week test drive workouts in Chapter 9, no matter which of the Push, Pull, Swing tools you choose, you'll notice that each routine is made up of all five types of moves.

- ▶ One **upper body push** exercise
- ▶ One **upper body pull** exercise
- ▶ One **lower body push** exercise
- ▶ One **lower body pull** exercise
- ▶ One **swing** (rotational) or **core** exercise

Building your own Push, Pull, Swing routine isn't difficult. Think of it as a checklist—one that helps you quickly determine whether or not your workout is balanced. Here are some templates for various standard workouts to get you started.

REMEMBER THE 1-REP RULE

Always go 1 rep short of failure. Pushing, pulling, or swinging a weight to the point where you can't complete a solid repetition will burn your muscles out before the workout is over. It's critical that your body's central nervous system is able to recover after each workout to prevent overtraining. By leaving 1 rep "on the table" in every set, you'll still stimulate all of your muscle fibers without risking having to cut your workouts short—or worse, suffering an injury—due to overtraining.

Beginner 3-Day Workout

This follows a classic strength training format of three workouts a week with rest days in between workouts. Be sure to choose different push, pull, and swing exercises for each day (labeled A, B, and C exercises below).

DAY 1	DAY 2	DAY 3
Upper body push exercise A	Upper body push exercise B	Upper body push exercise C
Lower body push exercise A	Lower body push exercise B	Lower body push exercise C
Upper body pull exercise A	Upper body pull exercise B	Upper body pull exercise C
Lower body pull exercise A	Lower body pull exercise B	Lower body pull exercise C
Swing (rotational) or core exercise A	Swing (rotational) or core exercise B	Swing (rotational) or core exercise C

Intermediate 3-Day Workout

This workout separates the pushing and pulling upper body exercises and combines pushing and pulling for your lower body on the third day for the more advanced lifter who needs more work on his upper body muscles. This routine could be performed three times a week with a day of rest in between each workout or by lifting 3 days straight, resting 1 day, and then lifting another 3 days straight because you are working opposing muscle groups on Days 1 and 2. On Day 3, you can either repeat the swing or core exercises from Day 1 or choose two new ones.

DAY 1	DAY 2	DAY 3
Upper body push exercise A	Upper body pull exercise A	Lower body push exercise A
Upper body push exercise B	Upper body pull exercise B	Lower body pull exercise A
Upper body push exercise C	Upper body pull exercise C	Lower body push exercise B
Upper body push exercise D	Upper body pull exercise D	Lower body pull exercise B
Swing (rotational) or core exercise A	Swing (rotational) or core exercise C	Swing (rotational) or core exercise A
Swing (rotational) or core exercise B	Swing (rotational) or core exercise D	Swing (rotational) or core exercise B

Intermediate 4-Day Workout

In this plan, you exercise 4 days a week with a day of rest in the middle. In each workout, you hit every muscle group, utilizing all pull moves for upper and lower body one day, all push moves for upper and lower body another, and incorporating swing moves into both days. For the second pair of days, you can repeat the same first two workouts or select different exercises.

DAY 1	DAY 2	REST DAY	DAY 3	DAY 4
Upper body push exercise A	Upper body pull exercise A		Upper body push exercise A	Upper body pull exercise A
Lower body push exercise A	Lower body pull exercise A		Lower body push exercise A	Lower body pull exercise A
Upper body push exercise B	Upper body pull exercise B		Upper body push exercise B	Upper body pull exercise B
Lower body push exercise B	Lower body pull exercise B		Lower body push exercise B	Lower body pull exercise B
Upper body push exercise C	Upper body pull exercise C		Upper body push exercise C	Upper body pull exercise C
Lower body push exercise C	Lower body pull exercise C		Lower body push exercise C	Lower body pull exercise C
Swing (rotational) or core exercise A	Swing (rotational) or core exercise B		Swing (rotational) or core exercise C	Swing (rotational) or core exercise D

EXERCISE TYPE CHEAT SHEET

Is that a push, pull, or swing? To use the previous workout charts, it's helpful to have a list that organizes exercises by type (push, pull, swing) and tool, starting with dumbbells below. Here and on the next two pages are such lists to help you create balanced routines.

DUMBBELLS

UPPER BODY PUSH EXERCISES

CHEST PRESS (page 48)
Floor Press (page 49)
Incline Chest Press
  (page 49)
Alternating Chest Press
  (page 49)

CLEAN AND PRESS
(page 52)

**LYING TRICEPS
EXTENSION** (page 80)
Tate Press (page 80)

PUSHUP (page 66)
T-Pushup (page 67)
Pushup Drag (page 67)

**SINGLE-ARM TRICEPS
KICKBACK** (page 81)
Two-Arm Triceps Kickback
  (page 81)

**STANDING SHOULDER
PRESS** (page 84)
Single-Arm Shoulder Press
  (page 84)

UPPER BODY PULL EXERCISES

BICEPS CURL (page 46)
Incline Hammer Curl
  (page 47)
Zottman Curl (page 47)
Prone Hammer Curl
  (page 47)

CHEST FLY (page 50)
Incline Chest Fly (page 50)

CLEAN AND PRESS
(page 52)

LATERAL RAISE (page 60)
Seated (or Kneeling)
  Lateral Raise (page 61)
Lateral T-Raise (page 61)
Single-Arm Lateral Raise
  (page 61)

PULLOVER (page 83)
Cross-Bench Pullover
  (page 83)

REAR LATERAL RAISE
(page 62)

SHRUG (page 69)

BENT-OVER ROW
(page 77)
Lawnmower Pull (page 77)

TWO-ARM ROW (page 76)
Single-Leg Row (page 76)

LOWER BODY PUSH EXERCISES

FRONT SQUAT (page 53)

LUNGE (page 64)
Walking Lunge (page 65)
Side Lunge (page 65)

SQUAT (page 54)
Jump Squat (page 55)
Bulgarian Isometric Squat
  (page 55)

STEPUP (page 74)
Crossover Stepup
  (page 75)

**SINGLE-LEG STANDING
CALF RAISE** (page 63)

LOWER BODY PULL EXERCISES

CLEAN AND PRESS
(page 52)

DEADLIFT (page 56)
Neutral-Grip Deadlift
  (page 57)
Sumo Deadlift (page 57)

HIGH PULL (page 112)

ROMANIAN DEADLIFT
(page 58)
Single-Leg Romanian
  Deadlift (page 58)

SNATCH (page 86)

**STRAIGHT-LEG
DEADLIFT** (page 59)
Single-Leg Straight-Leg
  Deadlift (page 59)

SWING (AND CORE) EXERCISES

CRUNCH (page 51)
Long-Arm Crunch (page 51)

REVERSE CRUNCH (page 70)
Double Crunch (page 70)

KNEELING TWIST (page 71)
Russian Twist (page 71)

SIDE PLANK (page 72)

STANDING TWIST (page 73)

WOODCHOP (page 78)
Single-Leg Woodchop (page 79)
Reverse Woodchop (page 79)

Refer to the list on page 87 for additional exercises that can also be performed using a dumbbell.

(continued)

EXERCISE TYPE CHEAT SHEET (*cont.*)

KETTLEBELL

UPPER BODY PUSH EXERCISES

CLEAN (page 90)

CLEAN AND PRESS
(page 92)
Double Clean and Press
(page 93)

PUSHUP (page 114)
Pushup Drag (page 115)
Death Crawl (page 115)

**SINGLE-ARM PUSH
PRESS** (page 120)
Two-Arm Push Press
(page 120)

SHOULDER PRESS
(page 118)
Two-Hand Shoulder Press
(page 119)
Seesaw Press (page 119)
Bottom-Up Shoulder Press
(page 119)

SOTS PRESS (page 121)

UPPER BODY PULL EXERCISES

BENT-OVER ROW
(page 98)
45-Degree Two-Arm Row
(page 99)
Yates Row (page 99)
Single-Leg Row (page 99)

IRON CROSS (page 117)

RENEGADE ROW
(page 130)
Renegade Row and Burpee
(page 131)

LOWER BODY PUSH EXERCISES

FARMER'S WALK
(page 102)
Suitcase Carry (page 103)
Rack Walk (page 103)
Overhead Farmer's Walk
(page 103)

GOBLET SQUAT
(page 126)
Wide-Stance Goblet Squat
(page 127)
Thruster (page 127)

PISTOL SQUAT (page 128)

REVERSE LUNGE
(page 122)
Overhead Lunge
(page 123)
Goblet Lunge (page 123)

TACTICAL LUNGE
(page 124)

TURKISH GETUP
(page 132)
Half-Getup (page 133)

LOWER BODY PULL EXERCISES

CLEAN (page 90)
Hang Clean (page 91)
Dead Clean (page 91)
Double Clean (page 90)

CLEAN AND PRESS
(page 92)
Double Clean and Press
(page 93)

DEADLIFT (page 97)
Double Deadlift (page 97)

HIGH PULL (page 112)
Double High Pull (page 113)
One-Arm High Pull
(page 113)

ROMANIAN DEADLIFT
(page 100)
Single-Leg Romanian
Deadlift (page 100)

SNATCH (page 110)
Two-Hand Snatch
(page 111)

SINGLE-ARM SWING
(page 106)
Alternating Single-Arm
Swing (page 107)

DOUBLE-ARM SWING
(page 108)
Walking Swing (page 109)
Half-Turn Swing (page 109)
Double Swing (page 109)

SWING (AND CORE) EXERCISES

AROUND-THE-BODY PASS (page 94)
Around-the-Legs Pass (page 95)

HALO (page 116)

BENT PRESS (page 101)

FIGURE-EIGHT (page 96)

WINDMILL (page 134)
Double Windmill (page 135)

Refer to the chart on page 135 for additional exercises that can also be performed using a kettlebell.

SANDBAG

UPPER BODY PUSH EXERCISES

LATERAL DRAG
(page 182)

PUSHUP (page 170)

CLEAN AND PRESS
(page 158)
Staggered Stance Clean
and Press (page 158)

SHOULDER-TO-SHOULDER PRESS
(page 178)
Kneeling Shoulder-to-
Shoulder Press (page 179)
Staggered Stance Shoulder-
to-Shoulder Press
(page 179)
Side Lunge/Shoulder-to-
Shoulder Press (page 179)

UPPER BODY PULL EXERCISES

LATERAL DRAG
(page 182)

SINGLE-LEG ROW
(page 180)
Vertical Single-Leg Row
(page 181)
Neutral-Grip Bent-Over Row
(page 181)
Staggered Stance Bent-
Over Row (page 181)

SHOULDERING
(page 142)
One-Arm Shouldering
(page 143)
Side Lunge Shouldering
(page 143)

LOWER BODY PUSH EXERCISES

BEAR HUG SQUAT
(page 139)
Wide-Stance Bear Hug
Squat (page 139)

ROTATING LUNGE
(page 156)
Alternating Rotating Lunge
(page 157)
Rotating Lunge Clean
(page 157)

DRAG (page 160)
Offset Drag (page 161)
One-Arm Drag (page 161)

FARMER'S WALK
(page 162)
Offset Farmer's Walk
(page 163)
Bear Hug Farmer's Walk
(page 163)
Overhead Farmer's Walk
(page 163)
One-Arm Overhead Farm-
er's Walk (page 163)

GETUP (page 164)
Side Crunch Hip Thrust
(page 165)
Bottom-Half Getup
(page 165)

TURKISH GETUP
(page 166)

REVERSE LUNGE
(page 172)
Clean and Lunge
(page 173)
Rotational Reverse Lunge
(page 173)

SIDE LUNGE (page 174)
Side Lunge Deadlift
(page 175)
Side Lunge Clean
(page 175)

ZERCHER SQUAT
(page 145)
Zercher Squat and Press
(page 145)

LOWER BODY PULL EXERCISES

ROTATING CLEAN
(page 148)
Rotating Clean and Press
(page 149)
Rotating Clean Lunge Press
(page 149)

ROTATING DEADLIFT
(page 150)
Alternating Rotating Deadlift
(page 151)

SHOVELING (page 152)

SHUCKING (page 153)

ROTATING HANG PULL
(page 154)
Rotating High Pull
(page 154)

BEAR HUG (page 138)

CLEAN (page 140)

GOOD MORNING
(page 168)
Good Morning Front Squat
(page 169)
Bear Hug Good Morning
(page 169)
Single-Leg Good Morning
(page 169)

SHOULDERING (page 142)
One-Arm Shouldering
(page 143)
Side Lunge Shouldering
(page 143)

SNATCH (page 144)
Rotating Snatch (page 144)

SWING (page 176)
Single-Arm Swing
(page 176)

SWING (AND CORE) EXERCISES

LONG-ARM CRUNCH (page 146)
Standard Crunch (page 147)
Overhead Raise Long-Arm Crunch (page 147)

AROUND-THE-WORLD (page 155)

WIPER (page 177)

SIDE-TO-SIDE PICKUP (page 171)

Refer to the lists on page 183 for additional exercises that can be performed using a sandbag.

Points to Keep in Mind

As simple as getting fit by pushing, pulling, and swinging is, it is not an exact science. These principles will help you avoid confusion.

1 **NOT ALL EXERCISES ARE CREATED EQUAL.** Although each exercise is grouped by type (pushing, pulling, or swinging), some exercises—because of tweaks, such as adding a lunging, pressing, or twisting motion—actually fit into several categories.

For example, you'll find the Rotating Clean Lunge Press—a variation of a Rotating Clean—on the lower body pulling exercise. However, having to lunge as well as press the sandbag overhead adds a pushing element to the exercise. What's more, you also rotate and swing the sandbag. So, in reality, this exercise is a push, pull, and swing exercise. Don't sweat it. Just go with the flow. We categorize the exercises according to the majority of the muscles used in the movement.

2 **A FEW EXERCISES ARE LISTED IN SEVERAL CATEGORIES.** Certain moves are such a complete body effort that it would be unfair to have to flip a coin to decide which category they belong in.

For example, the Clean and Press is an effective lower body pulling exercise, but it is equally impressive as an upper body pushing exercise. With movements that are a 50-50 split in terms of effort, you'll find them listed twice in separate categories.

3 **WHEN IN DOUBT, TRUST YOUR BODY.** As you experiment with the moves in this book, you'll notice which exercises can be considered more than just one type of movement. For instance, you may get a great core workout from an exercise that you thought was merely a pulling exercise.

So if some exercises can be considered more than one type of exercise, how exactly are you supposed to create a balanced workout? That's easy. As you create your workouts, try this trick: First, write down these five categories.

- ▶ **Upper body push** exercise
- ▶ **Upper body pull** exercise
- ▶ **Lower body push** exercise
- ▶ **Lower body pull** exercise
- ▶ **Swing** (rotational) or **core** exercise

Next, run through every exercise in your routine, then check off which category (or categories) each exercise seems to fulfill. Once you've run through all the exercises, count them up and see what type of ratio you're dealing with, and yes, count an exercise twice (or more) if it falls into multiple categories to get an accurate sense of your routine.

Do the math—but please don't hang yourself by it. This is not an exact science, as I mentioned before. It's intended to be a second set of eyes to make sure you're training your body the way it was meant to be trained—head to toe, back to front, and everything in between. It's a smarter, simpler solution to give you peace of mind that the hours you spend exercising each week are getting maximum results for you. You can use it, or you can use each exercise in this book in any way that you choose, in any type of routine that you choose. But don't feel as if you have to create a workout that is the perfect balance every single time.

THE BASICS OF MUSCLE BUILDING

1 **Work large body parts before small body parts.** That means you should select exercises that primarily work your big muscle groups first. If you have time during your workouts, you may add in exercises that target smaller muscles (such as your triceps, biceps, calves, and abs).

Another way to organize workouts if you want more bang for your buck: Choose compound exercises over single-joint exercises. For example, pick exercises like Squats over Calf Raises, Chest Presses over Chest Flies, Clean and Presses over Lateral Raises, and Bent-Over Rows over Biceps Curls.

Most experts agree that the first exercise in each workout should be the one that requires the most effort. That way, you're performing the hardest exercises while your muscles are fresh and your energy levels are at their highest.

2 **Know the right numbers.** How many exercises you should put into a routine, how many sets you should perform of each exercise, how many reps you should perform of each exercise, and how long you should rest between sets—all of these depend on your fitness goals. The following chart is a guideline that makes it a little easier to figure out what to do. These aren't magic numbers, mind you, but they are a good benchmark for most men, most of the time.

GOAL	TOTAL EXERCISES	NUMBER OF SETS	REPS	REST INTERVAL BETWEEN SETS
Muscle strength and power	3–5	4–6 (chest, back, legs)	3–5	3–4 minutes
		2–3 accessory muscle groups (shoulders, arms, core)	8–10	1–2 minutes
Maximum muscle hypertrophy	6–8	3–4	6–12	1–2 minutes
Maximum fat loss	8–10	1–2	8–15	0–30 seconds

Basically, your set count should be inversely related to your number of reps per set. That means that if you're performing a high number of reps (such as 12 to 15), 1 or 2 sets should be enough. For 10 to 12 reps, try 2 or 3 sets. For 8 reps, 3 or 4 sets would work well. And if you're doing 3 to 5 reps per set, you probably want to do 4 to 6 sets.

3 **Keep it under four workouts per week and 60 minutes per workout.** Any more than 4 days is too much, unless you're an elite athlete with several years' experience behind you. Otherwise, your muscles will never have enough time to recover—and you won't see as many, if any, gains. After that threshold, results dwindle and injury risk increases.

That also goes for how long you exercise. Your body reduces its production of muscle-building hormones and elevates its production of muscle-wasting hormones at about the 60-minute mark. Keeping your workouts intense but brief will yield much better results than shooting for a marathon workout.

4 **Say good-bye to your workout after 4 to 6 weeks.** Your workouts will turn boring—even counterproductive—if you don't revise them after that time. In order to keep your muscles interested and evolving, come up with something new, even if it's just a change in reps, sets, or rest intervals. Or try switching your usual fitness tool for one of the other two.

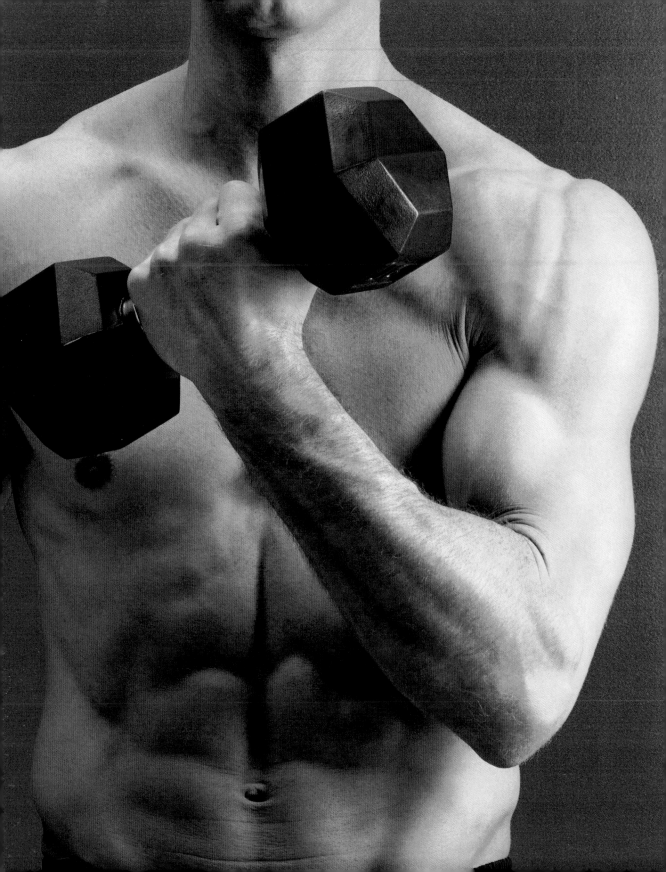

11

THE WORKOUTS

11 TOP TRAINERS' PROGRAMS FOR DUMBBELLS, KETTLEBELLS, AND SANDBAGS

There's something about having a well-thought-out plan that makes any goal easier to reach. That's what this chapter delivers: Think of it as a series of to-do lists for achieving the body and fitness level you want.

On the following pages, you'll find premade plans for Push, Pull, Swing workouts choreographed by expert trainers who've been preaching the gospel of multiplanar training with dumbbells, kettlebells, and sandbags for many years and with great success.

You'll find workouts designed to help you boost fat loss, build muscle, and improve athletic performance with each specific piece of gear. Since you probably have experience with dumbbells, we'll kickstart with two dynamic

workouts—the Kettlebell Shredder and the Sandstorm—that will help you get comfortable with the less-familiar equipment.

Each of the workouts in this chapter is designed by a different trainer, so you'll get a variety of unique perspectives. All the programs were built from the exercises described in Chapters 6, 7, and 8. Remember that in some cases where an exercise is performed basically the same way no matter which piece of equipment you use, its description may be found only once in either Chapter 6, 7, or 8. For example, the Biceps Curl is only found in the dumbbell chapter because it can be performed the same way using kettlebells or a sandbag. It's time to put these tools to work for you.

The Kettlebell Shredder

Because it is driven by the power of the totally athletic Hip Hinge movement, the kettlebell Swing is arguably among the most dynamic of total-body strength exercises. That's why it figures prominently in this extremely challenging 4-week workout from former weight-lifting champion Dan John.

John likes to say, "Focus on movements, not muscles." Isolating specific muscles, he says, "is training like you're Frankenstein's monster." Stiff. Mechanical. Lacking the fluidity of the human body. Instead, perform workouts loaded with compound, multijoint exercises that force your muscles to work as they were designed to in real life—and do a lot of repetitions.

This program combines elements of mobility, stability, strength, and cardio. That's why it's a 5-day-a-week routine made up of five different workouts, including a Tabata protocol done twice a month. (A Tabata is a version of a high-intesity interval workout pioneered by Japanese professor Izumi Tabata.) It delivers strength, sculpted muscles, and total-body functional fitness.

RULES TO REMEMBER

- Use this program for 4 weeks, 5 days a week, taking Thursdays and Sundays off as rest days.

- This program is made up of five different workouts: Simple Strength, Killer Cardio, Sweat Cyclone (Tabata done bimonthly), Tonic Recharge, and Mobility. Tonic Recharge is an active-recovery workout that your body will need after the prior workout's Tabatas.

- You'll find unique instructions for each of the five workouts listed above each workout's chart. You'll notice that all but one of these workouts lack rest intervals. In most cases, the resistance exercises are paired with dynamic stretches, which serve as opportunities to catch your breath.

- Complete the five numbered workouts according to the chart shown on the opposite page.

- Always perform a comprehensive warmup before and cooldown after each workout.

ABOUT THE EXPERT

Dan John is an All-American discus thrower, strength coach, author, Fulbright Scholar, and online religious studies instructor. He has competed at the highest levels of Olympic weight lifting, as well as in the Highland Games and Weight Pentathlon, in which he holds an American record. A contributing writer for *Men's Health* magazine, he is the owner of the Westridge Street Barbell Club in Murray, Utah.

The 4-Week Plan

THE KETTLEBELL SHREDDER WEEKLY PLAN	MONDAY WORKOUT	TUESDAY WORKOUT	WEDNESDAY WORKOUT	FRIDAY WORKOUT	SATURDAY WORKOUT
Week 1	1	5	2	1	3
Week 2	4	5	1	2	1
Week 3	1	5	2	1	3
Week 4	4	5	1	2	1

Workout 1: Simple Strength

This workout pairs high-rep strength moves with dynamic stretches. Do each pair as a superset (back-to-back). Complete each superset three times without resting between them before moving to the next superset. Cap off your workout with the two "finishers" to boost your burn.

SIMPLE STRENGTH	STRENGTH	STRETCH
Superset 1	Single-Arm Push Press (page 120) (10 reps per arm)	Hip Flexor Stretch (page 105) (15 seconds per side)
Superset 2	Bent-Over Row (page 98) (10 reps per arm)	Hip Flexor Rainbow (page 105) (15 seconds per side)
Superset 3	Double-Arm Swing (page 108) (30 reps)	Bird Dog (page 104) (30 seconds, alternating legs)
Superset 4	Goblet Squat (page 126) (10 reps)	Six-Point Zenith (page 105) (30 seconds, alternating sides)
Finisher 1	Pushup-Position Plank (goal: 2 minutes) (page 105)	
Finisher 2	Suitcase Carry (page 103)	

Workout 2: Killer Cardio

This workout includes two strength moves: the Double-Arm Swing and the Goblet Squat, performed as a superset. Complete a total of 12 supersets. Between supersets, do a filler exercise for 30 seconds. Try to complete the workout without resting.

SUPERSET NUMBER	DOUBLE-ARM SWING/ GOBLET SQUAT SUPERSET	FILLER EXERCISE
1	15 swings / 1 squat	Hip Flexor Stretch (left foot forward) (page 105)
2	15 swings / 1 squat	Hip Flexor Stretch (right foot forward)
3	15 swings / 1 squat	Hip Flexor Rainbow (left foot forward) (page 105)
4	15 swings / 1 squat	Hip Flexor Rainbow (right foot forward)
5	15 swings / 1 squat	Bird Dog (left arm, right leg) (page 104)
6	15 swings / 1 squat	Bird Dog (right arm, left leg)
7	15 swings / 1 squat	Six-Point Zenith (right arm) (page 105)
8	15 swings / 1 squat	Six-Point Zenith (left arm)
9	15 swings / 1 squat	Pushup-Position Plank (page 105)
10	15 swings / 1 squat	Suitcase Carry (right hand) (page 103)
11	15 swings / 1 squat	Suitcase Carry (left hand)

Workout 3: Sweat Cyclone

You will do these two Tabatas only twice a month. See "The 4-Week Plan" on page 205. Do Tabata 2 immediately after completing 4 minutes of Tabata 1. You only get 10 seconds to rest, so be in position and ready to go at 7 seconds.

TABATA NUMBER	COMBINATION	TOTAL TIME
1	Goblet Squat (page 126) (20 seconds)/Rest (10 seconds)	4 minutes
2	Double-Arm Swing (page 108) (20 seconds)/Rest (10 seconds)	4 minutes

Workout 4: Tonic Recharge

Follow the instructions for Workout 1: Simple Strength, but use slightly lighter weights and complete just 1 set of each exercise.

SIMPLE STRENGTH	STRENGTH	STRETCH
Superset 1	Single-Arm Push Press (page 120) (10 reps per arm)	Hip Flexor Stretch (page 105) (15 seconds per side)
Superset 2	Bent-Over Row (supported) (page 98) (10 reps per arm)	Hip Flexor Rainbow (page 105) (15 seconds per side)
Superset 3	Double-Arm Swing (page 108) (30 reps)	Bird Dog (page 104) (30 seconds, alternating legs)
Superset 4	Goblet Squat (page 126) (10 reps)	Six-Point Zenith (page 105) (30 seconds, alternating sides)
Finisher 1	Pushup-Position Plank (page 105) (goal: 2 minutes)	
Finisher 2	Suitcase Carry (page 103)	

Workout 5: Mobility

Do 3 circuits of the following stretches without pausing to rest.

STRETCH	DURATION
Hip Flexor (page 105)	30 seconds per side
Hip Flexor Rainbow (page 105)	30 seconds per side
Bird Dog (page 104)	30 seconds per side
Six-Point Zenith (page 105)	30 seconds per side

The Sandstorm

Two herniated discs ended Josh Henkin's college basketball days, and after physical therapy he needed a way to retrain the movements he had avoided due to pain.

"Basically, the sandbag helped me reeducate my body to move properly," says Henkin, now a certified strength and conditioning specialist who has built a business around sandbag training. "The sandbag's shape shifts, creating an unstable load that forces muscles to work together to keep balance." What's more, the constant rebalancing challenge creates metabolic turbulence—or you might call it a sandstorm—that burns calories before and after your workout.

The unique shape of a sandbag and its instability allow you to perform a far greater variety of moves than you would be able to with traditional bar weights. There are two basic ways to increase the level of difficulty of your sandbag workout—by holding the bag differently and by changing how you stand when you perform an exercise. For example, by using a staggered stance or by stepping to the side, you can increase the stability demands of an exercise. And holding the bag horizontally above your head rather than vertically at your chest will challenge your core differently during certain moves. "It's easy to add many layers of complexity to an exercise," says Henkin.

RULES TO REMEMBER

- Use this plan for 4 weeks, 3 days a week, taking at least 48 hours to recover in between workouts.

- Do the program in circuit style. Repeat the circuit for the complete number of sets.

- Exercises identified with the same number and different letters should be performed by alternating back and forth between sets of the exercises as many times as possible for the time listed. Take only as much rest as needed in between to complete quality reps. The goal is to see how many rounds you can do within the given time. The remaining exercises in the workout should be done as a circuit.

- Intermediate exercisers use 50 to 60 pounds as a base and a lighter weight of 30 pounds for more complex moves. Advanced exercisers can use 70 to 80 pounds as a base and a lighter weight of 35 pounds.

ABOUT THE EXPERT

Josh Henkin, CSCS, is the creator and CEO of Ultimate Sandbag Training (ultimatesandbagtraining.com). His program has been featured in magazines, on network programs, and at fitness conferences worldwide. Henkin was also commissioned by the US Army Special Forces Recruiting Battalion to develop a fitness program that could be performed anytime, anywhere.

WEEK 1

Workout 1

EXERCISES	SETS	REPS	REST
1A. Rotating Lunge (page 156)	As many as possible in 10 minutes	10 per side	As little as necessary
1B. Neutral-Grip Bent-Over Row (page 181)		6	As little as necessary
Clean and Press (page 158)	3	6–8	30 seconds
Around-the-World (page 155)	3	12–15 per side	30 seconds
Grip Curl (page 159)	3	8–10	30 seconds

Workout 2

EXERCISES	SETS	REPS	REST
1A. Good Morning (page 168)	As many as possible in 10 minutes	12	As little as necessary
1B. Kneeling Shoulder-to-Shoulder Press (Arc Press) (page 179)		6 per side	As little as necessary
Bear Hug Squat (page 139)	3	10–12	30 seconds
Staggered Stance Bent-Over Row (page 181)	3	6–8 per side	30 seconds
Rotating High Pull (page 154)	3	10–12 per side	30 seconds

Workout 3

EXERCISES	SETS	REPS	REST
1A. Front Squat (page 53)	As many as possible in 10 minutes	10 per side	As little as necessary
1B. Rotating Clean (page 148)		8 per side	As little as necessary
Neutral-Grip Bent-Over Row (page 181)	3	10–12	30 seconds
Bottom-Half Getup (also called Shoulder Leg Threading) (page 165)	3	5–6 per side	30 seconds
Shucking (page 153)	3	8–10 per side	30 seconds

WEEK 2

Workout 1

EXERCISES	SETS	REPS	REST
Rotating Lunge (page 156)	3	As many as possible in 30 seconds	30 seconds
Neutral-Grip Bent-Over Row (page 181)	3	As many as possible in 30 seconds	30 seconds
Clean and Press (page 158)	3	As many as possible in 30 seconds	30 seconds
Around-the-World (page 155)	3	As many as possible in 30 seconds per side	30 seconds
Grip Curl (page 159)	3	As many as possible in 30 seconds	30 seconds

Workout 2

EXERCISES	SETS	REPS	REST
Good Morning (page 168)	3	As many as possible in 30 seconds	30 seconds
Kneeling Shoulder-to-Shoulder Press (Arc Press) (page 179)	3	As many as possible in 30 seconds	30 seconds
Bear Hug Squat (page 139)	3	As many as possible in 30 seconds	30 seconds
Staggered Stance Bent-Over Row (page 181)	3	As many as possible in 30 seconds per foot position	30 seconds in between and after second foot position
Rotating Hang Pull (page 154)	3	As many as possible in 30 seconds	30 seconds

Workout 3

EXERCISES	SETS	REPS	REST
Front Squat (page 53)	3	As many as possible in 30 seconds	30 seconds
Rotating Clean (page 148)	3	As many as possible in 30 seconds	30 seconds
Neutral-Grip Bent-Over Row (page 181)	3	As many as possible in 30 seconds	30 seconds
Bottom-Half Getup (also called Shoulder Leg Threading) (page 165)	3	30 seconds per side	no rest between sides 30 seconds
Shucking (page 153)	3	As many as possible in 30 seconds	30 seconds

WEEK 3

Workout 1

EXERCISES	SETS	REPS	REST
1A. Rotating Lunge (page 156)	As many as possible in 15 minutes	10 per side	As little as necessary
1B. Neutral-Grip Bent-Over Row (page 181)		6	As little as necessary
2A. Clean and Press (page 158)	3	8–10	30 seconds
2B. Around-the-World (page 155)	2	10–12 per side	30 seconds
2C. Grip Curl (page 159)	2	10–12	30 seconds

Workout 2

EXERCISES	SETS	REPS	REST
1A. Good Morning (page 168)	As many as possible in 15 minutes	12	As little as necessary
1B. Kneeling Shoulder-to-Shoulder Press (Arc Press) (page 179)		8 per side	As little as necessary
Bear Hug Squat (page 139)	3	8–10, with a 2-second pause at bottom	30 seconds
Staggered Stance Bent-Over Row (page 181)	3	8–10 per side	30 seconds
Rotating Hang Pull (page 154)	3	8–10 per side	30 seconds

Workout 3

EXERCISES	SETS	REPS	REST
1A. Front Squat (page 53)	As many as possible in 15 minutes	10 per side	As little as necessary
1B. Rotating Clean (page 148)		6 per side	As little as necessary
Neutral-Grip Bent-Over Row (page 181)	3	10–12 with pause at top	30 seconds
Bottom-Half Getup (also called Shoulder Leg Threading) (page 165)	3	6 per side	30 seconds
Shucking (page 153)	3	12–15 per side	30 seconds

WEEK 4

Workout 1

EXERCISES	SETS	REPS	REST
Rotating Lunge (page 156)	3	As many as possible in 40 seconds	20 seconds
Neutral-Grip Bent-Over Row (page 181)	3	As many as possible in 40 seconds	20 seconds
Clean and Press (page 158)	3	As many as possible in 40 seconds	20 seconds
Around-the-World (page 155)	3	As many as possible in 40 seconds per direction	20 seconds between directions
Grip Curl (page 159)	3	As many as possible in 40 seconds	20 seconds

Workout 2

EXERCISES	SETS	REPS	REST
Good Morning (page 168)	3	As many as possible in 40 seconds	20 seconds
Kneeling Shoulder-to-Shoulder Press (Arc Press) (page 179)	3	As many as possible in 40 seconds	20 seconds
Bear Hug Squat (page 139)	3	As many as possible in 40 seconds	20 seconds
Staggered Stance Bent-Over Row (page 181)	3	As many as possible in 40 seconds per side	20 seconds between sides and after second side
Rotating Hang Pull (page 154)	3	As many as possible in 40 seconds	20 seconds

Workout 3

EXERCISES	SETS	REPS	REST
Front Squat (page 53)	3	As many as possible in 40 seconds	20 seconds
Rotating Clean (page 148)	3	As many as possible in 40 seconds (alternating sides)	20 seconds
Neutral-Grip Bent-Over Row (page 181)	3	As many as possible in 40 seconds	20 seconds
Bottom-Half Getup (also called Shoulder Leg Threading) (page 165)	3	As many as possible in 40 seconds	20 seconds between sides and after second side
Shucking (page 153)	3	As many as possible in 40 seconds	20 seconds

Dumbbell Fat Blaster

If you're looking to burn off serious fat but only have access to dumbbells, this 4-week plan from personal trainer Brian Sutton challenges your muscles through every possible direction, improving your coordination and balance while it blasts away fat. "What makes dumbbells ideal for fat loss is how their versatility minimizes the boredom factor," says Sutton. "With an unlimited amount of exercise options, you have the ability in an instant to change course—without having to lower the intensity."

This workout combines some of the best compound exercises and multimuscle moves into a high-intensity program with a tempo that never gives your body a break, keeping your metabolism high from start to finish. Best of all, you'll notice a vast improvement in your posture, flexibility, muscular endurance, stamina, and strength, so your body won't simply be trim—it will be transformed.

RULES TO REMEMBER

- Use this plan for 4 weeks, 3 days a week, taking at least 48 hours to recover between workouts.

- Due to its intensity level, this workout is designed for intermediate to advanced exercisers. If you are a beginner, start with one of the workouts in Chapter 9 or 10.

- Exercises marked with the same number and either A or B are supersets, which should be performed back-to-back with no rest in between. After performing each superset, rest for the amount of time listed after the second exercise of the superset. Then repeat the cycle to complete the required supersets before moving to the next superset.

- For Workouts 2 and 3, complete all sets of each exercise, resting in between, then move to the next exercise.

- For any exercise that works one limb at a time, perform the exercise twice (once for each side) for the required repetitions before moving on.

ABOUT THE EXPERT

Brian Sutton, MS, MA, National Academy of Sports Medicine–certified personal trainer (NASM-CPT), is a corrective exercise and performance enhancement specialist and director of development for the NASM. He's also an adjunct faculty member for California University of Pennsylvania in the exercise science and sports studies department.

WEEK 1

Workout 1

EXERCISES	SETS	REPS	REST
1A. Front Squat (page 53)	2	12	None
1B. Single-Leg Romanian Deadlift (page 58)	2	12	60 seconds
2A. Incline Chest Press (page 49)	2	12	None
2B. T-Pushup (page 67)	2	12	60 seconds
3A. 45-Degree Two-Arm Row (page 99)	2	12	None
3B. Renegade Row (page 130)	2	12	60 seconds
4A. Standing Shoulder Press (page 84)	2	12	None
4B. Single-Arm Lateral Raise (page 61)	2	12	60 seconds
5A. Reverse Crunch (page 70)	2	12	None
5B. Side Plank (page 72)	2	12 (hold 3–5 seconds per rep)	60 seconds

Workout 2

EXERCISES	SETS	REPS	REST
Half Getup (page 133)	2	15	60 seconds
Goblet Lunge (page 123)	2	15	60 seconds
Single-Leg Straight-Leg Deadlift (page 59)	2	15	60 seconds
Pushup Drag (page 67)	2	15	60 seconds
Single-Leg Row (page 76)	2	15	60 seconds
Single-Arm Shoulder Press (page 84)	2	15	60 seconds
Zottman Curl (page 47)	2	15	60 seconds
Two-Arm Triceps Kickback (page 81)	2	15	60 seconds
Single-Leg Woodchop (page 79)	2	15	60 seconds
Windmill (page 134)	2	15	60 seconds

Workout 3

EXERCISES	SETS	REPS	REST
Clean and Press (page 52)	3	5	90 seconds
Snatch (page 86)	3	5	90 seconds
Push Press (page 68)	3	5	90 seconds
Deadlift (page 56)	3	8	90 seconds
Chest Press (page 48)	3	8	90 seconds
Pullover (page 83)	3	8	90 seconds
Shrug (page 69)	3	8	90 seconds

WEEK 2

Workout 1

EXERCISES	SETS	REPS	REST
1A. Front Squat (page 53)	3	8	None
1B. Single-Leg Romanian Deadlift (page 58)	3	8	60 seconds
2A. Incline Chest Press (page 49)	3	8	None
2B. T-Pushup (page 67)	3	8	60 seconds
3A. 45-Degree Two-Arm Row (page 99)	3	8	None
3B. Renegade Row (page 130)	3	8	60 seconds
4A. Standing Shoulder Press (page 84)	3	8	None
4B. Single-Arm Lateral Raise (page 61)	3	8	60 seconds
5A. Reverse Crunch (page 70)	3	8	None
5B. Side Plank (page 72)	3	8 (hold 3–5 seconds per rep)	60 seconds

Workout 2

EXERCISES	SETS	REPS	REST
Half Getup (page 133)	3	8	45 seconds
Goblet Lunge (page 123)	3	8	45 seconds
Single-Leg Straight-Leg Deadlift (page 59)	3	8	45 seconds
Pushup Drag (page 67)	3	8	45 seconds
Single-Leg Row (page 76)	3	8	45 seconds
Single-Arm Shoulder Press (page 84)	3	8	45 seconds
Zottman Curl (page 47)	3	8	45 seconds
Two-Arm Triceps Kickback (page 81)	3	8	45 seconds
Single-Leg Woodchop (page 79)	3	8	45 seconds
Windmill (page 134)	3	8	45 seconds

Workout 3

EXERCISES	SETS	REPS	REST
Clean and Press (page 52)	4	5	90 seconds
Snatch (page 86)	4	5	90 seconds
Push Press (page 68)	4	5	90 seconds
Deadlift (page 56)	4	8	90 seconds
Chest Press (page 48)	4	8	90 seconds
Pullover (page 83)	4	8	90 seconds
Shrug (page 69)	4	8	90 seconds

WEEK 3

Workout 1

EXERCISES	SETS	REPS	REST
1A. Front Squat (page 53)	3	10	None
1B. Single-Leg Romanian Deadlift (page 58)	3	10	60 seconds
2A. Incline Chest Press (page 49)	3	10	None
2B. T-Pushup (page 67)	3	10	60 seconds
3A. 45-Degree Two-Arm Row (page 99)	3	10	None
3B. Renegade Row (page 130)	3	10	60 seconds
4A. Standing Shoulder Press (page 84)	3	10	None
4B. Single-Arm Lateral Raise (page 61)	3	10	60 seconds
5A. Reverse Crunch (page 70)	3	10	None
5B. Side Plank (page 72)	3	10 (hold 3–5 seconds per rep)	60 seconds

Workout 2

EXERCISES	SETS	REPS	REST
Half Getup (page 133)	3	10	45 seconds
Goblet Lunge (page 123)	3	10	45 seconds
Single-Leg Straight-Leg Deadlift (page 59)	3	10	45 seconds
Pushup Drag (page 67)	3	10	45 seconds
Single-Leg Row (page 76)	3	10	45 seconds
Single-Arm Shoulder Press (page 84)	3	10	45 seconds
Zottman Curl (page 47)	3	10	45 seconds
Two-Arm Triceps Kickback (page 81)	3	10	45 seconds
Single-Leg Woodchop (page 79)	3	10	45 seconds
Windmill (page 134)	3	10	45 seconds

Workout 3

EXERCISES	SETS	REPS	REST
Clean and Press (page 52)	5	5	90 seconds
Snatch (page 86)	5	5	90 seconds
Push Press (page 68)	5	5	90 seconds
Deadlift (page 56)	5	8	90 seconds
Chest Press (page 48)	5	8	90 seconds
Pullover (page 83)	5	8	90 seconds
Shrug (page 69)	5	8	90 seconds

WEEK 4

Workout 1

EXERCISES	SETS	REPS	REST
1A. Front Squat (page 53)	3	12	None
1B. Single-Leg Romanian Deadlift (page 58)	3	12	60 seconds
2A. Incline Chest Press (page 49)	3	12	None
2B. T-Pushup (page 67)	3	12	60 seconds
3A. 45-Degree Two-Arm Row (page 99)	3	12	None
3B. Renegade Row (page 130)	3	12	60 seconds
4A. Standing Shoulder Press (page 84)	3	12	None
4B. Single-Arm Lateral Raise (page 61)	3	12	60 seconds
5A. Reverse Crunch (page 70)	3	12	None
5B. Side Plank (page 72)	3	12 (hold 3–5 seconds per rep)	60 seconds

Workout 2

EXERCISES	SETS	REPS	REST
Half Getup (page 133)	4	12	30 seconds
Goblet Lunge (page 123)	4	12	30 seconds
Single-Leg Straight-Leg Deadlift (page 59)	4	12	30 seconds
Pushup Drag (page 67)	4	12	30 seconds
Single-Leg Row (page 76)	4	12	30 seconds
Single-Arm Shoulder Press (page 84)	4	12	30 seconds
Zottman Curl (page 47)	4	12	30 seconds
Two-Arm Triceps Kickback (page 81)	4	12	30 seconds
Single-Leg Woodchop (page 79)	4	12	30 seconds
Windmill (page 134)	4	12	30 seconds

Workout 3

EXERCISES	SETS	REPS	REST
Clean and Press (page 52)	5	5	90 seconds
Snatch (page 86)	5	5	90 seconds
Push Press (page 68)	5	5	90 seconds
Deadlift (page 56)	5	8	90 seconds
Chest Press (page 48)	5	8	90 seconds
Pullover (page 83)	5	8	90 seconds
Shrug (page 69)	5	8	90 seconds

Kettlebell Fat Blaster

According to Eric Salvador, NASM-CPT, the most effective kettlebell fat-burning program must contain strength training movements that hit multiple muscle groups *and* some form of high-intensity interval training (HIIT). The HIIT here is a Kettlebell Swing done Tabata style. (A Tabata is a version of a high-intesity interval workout pioneered by Japanese professor Izumi Tabata.) This 4-week routine delivers both, adjusting the work-to-rest ratio each week as your body becomes acclimated and requires less time to recover from the intensity. It's a one-two punch that elevates your EPOC (excess post-exercise oxygen consumption), more commonly referred to as the "afterburn," a metabolism boost that could keep your body burning fat at a higher rate for as long as 48 hours after your workout.

RULES TO REMEMBER

- Use this plan for 4 weeks, 3 days a week, taking at least 48 hours to recover between workouts.

- On Days 1 and 2, perform each exercise for the required number of sets before moving on to the next exercise.

- The weight used for the Single-Arm Shoulder Press should be heavier than that used for the Two-Hand Shoulder Press.

- After the strength exercises, perform a 4-minute Tabata-style routine. Do the exercise as quickly as possible (while maintaining control of the weight) for 20 seconds, then rest for 10 seconds. Repeat eight times, for a total of 4 minutes.

- End each Day 1 and 2 workout with a finisher circuit. After completing the circuit, repeat it for the required number of rounds of the prescribed time.

- Day 3 is always a highly metabolic five-exercise circuit. You"ll do as many rounds as you can in 20 minutes.

ABOUT THE EXPERT

Eric Salvador is cocreator of the award-winning high-intensity training (HIT) class Ultimate Fitness Experience (UFX), taught throughout New York Sports Clubs, Philadelphia Sports Clubs, and Boston Sports Clubs, and he's the head instructor of the Fhitting Room in New York City.

WEEK 1			
DAY 1	**SETS**	**REPS**	**REST**
Shoulder Press (page 118)	3	10–12 each arm	60 seconds
Bent-Over Row (page 98)	3	10–12 each arm	60 seconds
Goblet Squat (page 126)	3	10–12	60 seconds
Lunge (page 64)	3	10–12	60 seconds
Windmill (page 134)	3	10–12 each side	60 seconds

Tabata:
Double-Arm Swing (20 seconds on/10 seconds off for 4 minutes) (page 108)

Finisher Circuit: Clean and Press (alternating sides) (page 92) Deadlift (page 97) Pushup (page 114) Crunch (kettlebell on chest) (page 51)	**Perform all four exercises, one after the other, for 30 seconds each, resting for 5 seconds between each exercise. Repeat the entire circuit twice, for a total of 3 circuits.**

DAY 2	**SETS**	**REPS**	**REST**
Single-Arm Push Press (page 120)	3	10–12 per arm	60 seconds
Bent-Over Row (page 98)	3	10–12	60 seconds
Front Squat (rack kettlebells by each shoulder) (page 53)	3	10–12 per side	60 seconds
Single-Leg Romanian Deadlift (page 100)	3	10–12 per leg	60 seconds
Half-Getup (page 133)	3	10–12 per arm	60 seconds

Tabata:
Figure-Eight (20 seconds on/10 seconds off for 4 minutes) (page 96)

Finisher Circuit: Hang Clean (page 91) Double-Arm Swing (page 108) Thruster (page 127) Russian Twist (page 71)	**Perform all four exercises, one after the other, for 30 seconds each, resting for 5 seconds between each exercise. For single-arm moves, use 15 seconds per arm. Repeat the entire circuit twice, for a total of 3 circuits.**

DAY 3	
Finisher Circuit: 10 Renegade Rows with Burpee (page 131) 10 Double Clean and Presses (page 93) 10 Front Squats (holding two kettlebells) (page 53) 10 Figure-Eights (page 96) 10 Double-Arm Swings (page 108)	**Perform all five exercises, one after the other, with no rest in between, for as many rounds as possible in 20 minutes.**

WEEK 2			
DAY 1	SETS	REPS	REST
Chest Press (page 48)	3	10–12	60 seconds
Halo (page 116)	3	10–12	60 seconds
Bent-Over Row (page 98)	3	10–12	60 seconds
Overhead Lunge (page 123)	3	10–12	60 seconds
Romanian Deadlift (page 100)	3	10–12	60 seconds
Turkish Getup (page 132)	3	10–12	60 seconds

Tabata:
Walking Swing (20 seconds on/10 seconds off for 4 minutes) (page 109)

Finisher Circuit: Alternating Single-Arm Swing (page 107) One-Arm High Pull (page 113) Seesaw Press (page 119) Tactical Lunge (page 124)	**Perform all four exercises, one after the other, for 45 seconds each, resting 10 seconds between each exercise. Repeat the entire circuit twice, for a total of 3 circuits.**

DAY 2	SETS	REPS	REST
Renegade Row (page 130)	3	10–12	60 seconds
Two-Hand Shoulder Press (page 119)	3	10–12	60 seconds
Lunge (page 64)	3	10–12 each leg	60 seconds
Double Windmill (page 135)	3	10–12	60 seconds

Tabata:
Double Clean (20 seconds on/10 seconds off for 4 minutes) (page 90)

Finisher Circuit: Thruster (page 127) Renegade Row with Burpee (page 131)	**Perform 20 reps of each exercise, then 15 reps each, then 10 reps each. Do not rest in between exercises or sets. Perform the circuit a total of three times.**

DAY 3	
Finisher Circuit: 10 Pistol Squats (5 per leg) (page 128) 10 Pushups (page 114) 15 Double-Arm Swings (page 108) Suitcase Carry (50 feet with each hand) (page 103)	**Perform all four exercises, one after the other, with no rest in between, for 10 rounds.**

WEEK 3			
DAY 1	SETS	REPS	REST
Double Clean and Press (page 93)	3	10–12	60 seconds
Single-Leg Row (page 99)	3	10–12 each side	60 seconds
Stepup (page 74)	3	10–12 each leg	60 seconds
Goblet Lunge (page 123)	3	10–12	60 seconds

Tabata:
Renegade Row and Burpee (20 seconds on/10 seconds off for 4 minutes) (page 131)

Finisher Circuit: Clean and Press (each arm) (page 92) Double Deadlift (page 97) Pushup (page 114)	Perform all three exercises, one after the other, for 60 seconds each, resting 30 seconds between each exercise. Repeat the entire circuit twice, for a total of 3 circuits.

DAY 2	SETS	REPS	REST
Two-Arm Push Press (page 120)	3	10–12	60 seconds
Bent-Over Row (page 98)	3	10–12	60 seconds
Front Squat (holding 2 kettlebells) (page 53)	3	10–12	60 seconds
Single-Leg Romanian Deadlift (page 100)	3	10–12 each leg	60 seconds
Rack Walk (page 103)	3	50 feet	60 seconds

Tabata:
Half-Turn Swing (20 seconds on/10 seconds off for 4 minutes) (page 109)

Finisher Circuit: Double Clean (page 90) Double-Arm Swing (page 108) Thruster (page 127) Russian Twist (page 71)	Perform all four exercises, one after the other, for 60 seconds each, resting 30 seconds between each exercise. Repeat the entire circuit twice, for a total of 3 circuits.

DAY 3

Finisher Circuit: 10 Renegade Rows with Burpee (page 131) 10 Double Clean and Presses (page 93) 10 Front Squats (holding 2 kettlebells) (page 53) 10 Figure-Eights (page 96) 10 Double-Arm Swings (page 108)	Perform all five exercises, one after the other, with no rest in between, for as many rounds as possible in 20 minutes.

WEEK 4			
DAY 1	SETS	REPS	REST
Chest Press (page 48)	3	10–12	60 seconds
Halo (from a lunge position) (page 116)	3	10–12	60 seconds
Side Lunge (page 65)	3	10–12 each leg	60 seconds
Romanian Deadlift (page 100)	3	10–12	60 seconds
Double Windmill (page 135)	3	10–12	60 seconds

Tabata:
Two-Hand Snatch (20 seconds on/10 seconds off for 4 minutes) (page 111)

Finisher Circuit: Alternating Single-Arm Swing (page 107) High Pull (page 112) Seesaw Press (seated) (page 119) Tactical Lunge (page 124)	Perform all four exercises, one after the other, for 60 seconds each, resting 30 seconds between each exercise. Repeat the entire circuit twice, for a total of 3 circuits.

DAY 2	SETS	REPS	REST
Chest Fly (page 50)	3	10–12	60 seconds
Dead Clean (page 91)	3	10–12	60 seconds
Deadlift (page 56)	3	10–12	60 seconds
Reverse Lunge (page 122)	3	10–12	60 seconds
Turkish Getup (page 132)	3	10–12	60 seconds

Tabata:
Double Clean (20 seconds on/10 seconds off for 4 minutes) (page 90)

Finisher Circuit: Thrusters (page 127) Renegade Row and Burpee (page 131)	Perform 20 reps of each exercise back-to-back, then 15 reps each, then 10 reps each, then 5 reps each. Do not rest in between exercises or sets. Perform the circuit a total of three times.

DAY 3

Finisher Circuit: 50 Double-Arm Swings (page 108) 40 Figure-Eights (page 96) 30 Double Cleans (page 90) 20 Kettlebell Pushups (page 114) 10 Front Squats (holding two kettlebells) (page 53)	Perform all five exercises, one after the other, with no rest in between. Rest for 2 minutes, then repeat the circuit twice, for a total of 3 circuits.

Sandbag Fat Blaster

"One of the biggest reasons most people fail to lose weight is that if a workout seems too complex, it's easy to find an excuse not to do it when your day starts to look too busy," says Annie Malaythong, personal trainer and fitness center owner. So she designed a simple 4-week circuit training program that yields superior results. It takes your body through a circuit of five multimuscle moves with no rest in between exercises and minimal rest between circuits, so it is perfect for people with limited time.

RULES TO REMEMBER

● Use this 3-workouts-per-week plan for 4 weeks. Perform Workouts 1, 2, and 3 each once a week, with an active rest day in between each workout and a full rest day at the end of each week. An active rest day includes any low-intensity exercise performed for 20 to 30 minutes at a pace that keeps your heart rate between 50 and 70 percent of your maximum.

● Each workout is a series of exercises performed as a circuit. After completing the circuit, rest for 2 minutes, then do 2 more circuits, resting for 2 minutes in between.

● Before and after each workout, do a session of self-myofascial release (SMR), or foam rolling.

● For any exercise that works one arm, leg, or side of your body at a time, perform the exercise twice (once for each side) for the required reps before moving to the next set or exercise.

ABOUT THE EXPERT

Annie Malaythong, NASM-CPT, PES, is a master instructor for the NASM, a mixed martial arts conditioning specialist, fitness nutrition specialist, Muay Thai practitioner, and owner of Studio 108, a fitness studio specializing in medical fitness in Johns Creek, Georgia. She was a fitness trainer on MTV's *I Used to Be Fat*.

WEEKS 1 THROUGH 4

Workout 1

EXERCISES	SETS	REPS
Clean and Press (page 158)	1	As many as possible in 30–45 seconds
Pushup (page 170)	1	As many as possible in 30–45 seconds
Bear Hug Good Morning (page 169)	1	As many as possible in 30–45 seconds
Reverse Woodchop (page 79)	1	As many as possible in 15 seconds per side
Push Press (page 68)	1	As many as possible in 30–45 seconds

Workout 2

EXERCISES	SETS	REPS
Single-Arm Swing (page 176)	1	As many as possible in 15 seconds per arm
Single-Leg Woodchop (page 79)	1	As many as possible in 15 seconds per leg
Single-Leg Good Morning (page 169)	1	As many as possible in 15 seconds per leg
Russian Twist (page 71)	1	As many as possible in 30–45 seconds
One-Arm Overhead Farmer's Walk (page 163)	1	As many as possible in 15 seconds per side

Workout 3

EXERCISES	SETS	REPS
Bear Hug Squat (page 139)	1	As many as possible in 30–45 seconds
Kneeling Shoulder-to-Shoulder Press (page 179)	1	As many as possible in 15 seconds per leg
Clean and Lunge (page 173)	1	As many as possible in 30–45 seconds
Shoulder-to-Shoulder Press (page 178)	1	As many as possible in 30–45 seconds
Side Lunge (page 174)	1	As many as possible in 30–45 seconds

Dumbbell Muscle Builder

If putting on as much muscle as possible is on your agenda, then this plan is for you. Created by Mike Fantigrassi, a 20-year veteran trainer, each workout starts with a power movement to activate your nervous system and uses varying rep ranges and loads to keep you progressing each week.

Fantigrassi also incorporates a simple technique that mixes horizontal loading (which basically means doing every set required of an exercise one right after the other) with vertical loading (doing 1 set of an exercise and then moving to the next exercise, until you've completed every exercise in the circuit before repeating the entire routine). "Most men tend to stick with one or the other for the length of a 4-, 6-, or 8-week program," says Fantigrassi. "By incorporating both into your workouts each week, your muscles are kept in a constant state of confusion that causes them to continuously adapt and grow."

RULES TO REMEMBER

- Use this plan for 4 weeks, 3 days a week, taking 48 hours to recover between workouts.

- On Day 1, you'll use compound movements and heavier loads, and you'll perform 1 set of each exercise before moving to the next exercise. After you finish the last exercise of the routine, you'll repeat the circuit.

- On Day 2, you'll use lighter weights and higher reps, but you'll complete every set for each exercise before moving to the next exercise.

- On Day 3, you'll use supersets. These exercises are marked with numbers and letters such as 1A, 1B and 2A, 2B that indicate moves that should be performed back-to-back, with no rest in between. You'll perform them in a circuit, so after you finish the last superset of the routine, you'll repeat the circuit.

ABOUT THE EXPERT

Mike Fantigrassi, MS, NASM-CPT, CSCS, is a master instructor at the National Academy of Sports Medicine. He has also worked as a certified personal trainer, nutrition coach, and metabolic technician.

WEEK 1

Workout 1

EXERCISES	SETS	REPS	REST
High Pull (page 112)	2	5 per arm	60 seconds
Deadlift (page 56)	2	8	60 seconds
Chest Press (page 48)	2	8	60 seconds
Pullover (page 83)	2	8	60 seconds
Push Press (page 68)	2	8	60 seconds
Long-Arm Crunch (page 51)	2	8	60 seconds

Rest for 3 minutes and repeat the circuit.

Workout 2

EXERCISES	SETS	REPS	REST
Snatch (page 86)	2	5	60 seconds
Stepup (page 74)	2	12 per leg, alternating	60 seconds
Chest Fly (page 50)	2	12	60 seconds
Bent-Over Row (page 77)	2	12 per arm	60 seconds
Lateral T-Raise (page 61)	2	12	60 seconds
Lying Triceps Extension (page 80)	2	12	60 seconds
Zottman Curl (page 47)	2	12	60 seconds
Single-Leg Standing Calf Raise (page 63)	2	12 per leg	60 seconds
Double Crunch (page 70)	2	12	None
Russian Twist (page 71)	2	12	30 seconds

Workout 3

EXERCISES	SETS	REPS	REST
1A. Double-Arm Swing (page 108)	2	12	None
1B. Romanian Deadlift (page 58)	2	12	60 seconds
2A. Incline Chest Press (page 49)	2	12	None
2B. Incline Chest Fly (page 50)	2	12	60 seconds
3A. 45-Degree Two-Arm Row (page 99)	2	12	None
3B. Rear Lateral Raise (page 62)	2	12	60 seconds
4A. Standing Shoulder Press (page 84)	2	12	None
4B. Tate Press (page 80)	2	12	None
4C. Zottman Curl (page 47)	2	12	60 seconds
5A. Reverse Crunch (page 70)	2	12	None
5B. Side Plank (page 72)	2	12 (hold 2–5 seconds per rep)	60 seconds

Rest 3 minutes and repeat the superset circuit.

WEEK 2

Workout 1

EXERCISES	SETS	REPS	REST
High Pull (page 112)	2	5 per arm	60 seconds
Deadlift (page 56)	2	6	60 seconds
Chest Press (page 48)	2	6	60 seconds
Pullover (page 83)	2	6	60 seconds
Push Press (page 68)	2	6	60 seconds
Long-Arm Crunch (page 51)	2	6	60 seconds

Rest for 3 minutes and repeat the circuit.

Workout 2

EXERCISES	SETS	REPS	REST
Snatch (page 86)	2	5	60 seconds
Stepup (page 74)	3	12 per leg, alternating	60 seconds
Chest Fly (page 50)	3	12	60 seconds
Bent-Over Row (page 77)	3	12 per arm	60 seconds
Lateral T-Raise (page 61)	3	12	60 seconds
Lying Triceps Extension (page 80)	3	12	60 seconds
Zottman Curl (page 47)	3	12	60 seconds
Single-Leg Standing Calf Raise (page 63)	3	12 per leg	60 seconds
Double Crunch (page 70)	3	12	None
Russian Twist (page 71)	3	12	30 seconds

Workout 3

EXERCISES	SETS	REPS	REST
1A. Double-Arm Swing (page 108)	2	10	None
1B. Romanian Deadlift (page 58)	2	10	60 seconds
2A. Incline Chest Press (page 49)	2	10	None
2B. Incline Chest Fly (page 50)	2	10	60 seconds
3A. 45-Degree Two-Arm Row (page 99)	2	10	None
3B. Rear Lateral Raise (page 62)	2	10	60 seconds
4A. Standing Shoulder Press (page 84)	2	10	None
4B. Tate Press (page 80)	2	10	None
4C. Zottman Curl (page 47)	2	10	60 seconds
5A. Reverse Crunch (page 70)	2	10	None
5B. Side Plank (page 72)	2	10 (hold 2–5 seconds per rep)	60 seconds

Rest 3 minutes and repeat the superset circuit.

WEEK 3

Workout 1

EXERCISES	SETS	REPS	REST
High Pull (page 112)	3	5 per arm	60 seconds
Deadlift (page 56)	3	8	60 seconds
Chest Press (page 48)	3	8	60 seconds
Pullover (page 83)	3	8	60 seconds
Push Press (page 68)	3	8	60 seconds
Long-Arm Crunch (page 51)	3	8	60 seconds

Rest for 3 minutes and repeat the circuit twice more.

Workout 2

EXERCISES	SETS	REPS	REST
Snatch (page 86)	2	5	60 seconds
Stepup (page 74)	2	10 per leg, alternating	60 seconds
Chest Fly (page 50)	2	10	60 seconds
Bent-Over Row (page 77)	2	10 per arm	60 seconds
Lateral T-Raise (page 61)	2	10	60 seconds
Lying Triceps Extension (page 80)	2	10	60 seconds
Zottman Curl (page 47)	2	10	60 seconds
Single-Leg Standing Calf Raise (page 63)	2	10 per leg	60 seconds
Double Crunch (page 70)	2	10	None
Russian Twist (page 71)	2	10	30 seconds

Workout 3

EXERCISES	SETS	REPS	REST
1A. Double-Arm Swing (page 108)	3	12	None
1B. Romanian Deadlift (page 58)	3	12	60 seconds
2A. Incline Chest Press (page 49)	3	12	None
2B. Incline Chest Fly (page 50)	3	12	60 seconds
3A. 45-Degree Two-Arm Row (page 99)	3	12	None
3B. Rear Lateral Raise (page 62)	3	12	60 seconds
4A. Standing Shoulder Press (page 84)	3	12	None
4B. Tate Press (page 80)	3	12	None
4C. Zottman Curl (page 47)	3	12	60 seconds
5A. Reverse Crunch (page 70)	3	12	None
5B. Side Plank (page 72)	3	12 (hold 2–5 seconds per rep)	60 seconds

Rest 3 minutes and repeat the superset twice more.

WEEK 4

Workout 1

EXERCISES	SETS	REPS	REST
High Pull (page 112)	3	5 per arm	60 seconds
Deadlift (page 56)	3	6	60 seconds
Chest Press (page 48)	3	6	60 seconds
Pullover (page 83)	3	6	60 seconds
Push Press (page 68)	3	6	60 seconds
Long-Arm Crunch (page 51)	3	6	60 seconds

Rest for 3 minutes and repeat the circuit twice more.

Workout 2

EXERCISES	SETS	REPS	REST
Snatch (page 86)	3	5	60 seconds
Stepup (page 74)	3	10 per leg, alternating	60 seconds
Chest Fly (page 50)	3	10	60 seconds
Bent-Over Row (page 77)	3	10 per arm	60 seconds
Lateral T-Raise (page 61)	3	10	60 seconds
Lying Triceps Extension (page 80)	3	10	60 seconds
Zottman Curl (page 47)	3	10	60 seconds
Single-Leg Standing Calf Raise (page 63)	3	10 per leg	60 seconds
Double Crunch (page 70)	3	10	None
Russian Twist (page 71)	3	10	30 seconds

Workout 3

EXERCISES	SETS	REPS	REST
1A. Double-Arm Swing (page 108)	3	10	None
1B. Romanian Deadlift (page 58)	3	10	60 seconds
2A. Incline Chest Press (page 49)	3	10	None
2B. Incline Chest Fly (page 50)	3	10	60 seconds
3A. 45-Degree Two-Arm Row (page 99)	3	10	None
3B. Rear Lateral Raise (page 62)	3	10	60 seconds
4A. Standing Shoulder Press (page 84)	3	10	None
4B. Tate Press (page 80)	3	10	None
4C. Zottman Curl (page 47)	3	10	60 seconds
5A. Reverse Crunch (page 70)	3	10	None
5B. Side Plank (page 72)	3	10 (hold 2–5 seconds per rep)	60 seconds

Rest 3 minutes and repeat the superset circuit twice more.

Kettlebell Muscle Builder

If you want to pack on major muscle, it takes maximum effort. That's why when we asked trainer Fabio Comana for a program that maximizes muscle size using only kettle-bells, he designed a program that optimizes metabolic stress in an effort to increase your hormonal response to build muscle. His workout uses techniques that include shorter recovery times (without compromising technique), more whole-body or compound lifts, and a large number of supersets and circuits to thoroughly engage and exhaust your entire body.

RULES TO REMEMBER

● Use this plan for 4 weeks, 4 days a week, taking at least 3 days to recover between sessions targeting the same muscle groups. That means you could follow a schedule such as Monday, lower body, Tues-day, upper body; Thursday, lower body, Friday, upper body.

● The goal is to maintain 10 to 12 reps for each portion of the set. If you can't do at least 10, then reduce the weight.

● Aim for a 4-second lowering phase with any exercise that is either a pull or a push.

● When you see a number with a letter next to it, such as 3A, it means that the exercise is to be performed as part of a superset. Do 1 set of the exercise, rest for the recommended amount of time, and then do 1 set of the next exercise in the group. Repeat until you've completed the required number of sets for each exercise in the superset.

ABOUT THE EXPERT

Fabio Comana, MA, MS, NASM-CPT, is a faculty instructor with the National Academy of Sports Medicine and a faculty member in exercise science and nutrition at San Diego State University and the University of California San Diego Extension.

WEEK 1

Workouts 1 and 3

EXERCISES	SETS	REPS	REST
1A. Standing Twist (warmup) (page 73)	1	As many as possible in 30 seconds	None
1B. Around-the-Body Pass (warmup) (page 94)	1	As many as possible in 30 seconds	None
1C. Halo (warmup) (page 116)	1	As many as possible in 30 seconds	None
1D. Single-Arm Swing (warmup) (page 106)	1	12 per arm	30 seconds
2A. Double Clean (page 90)	3	12	None
2B. Front Squat (page 53)		12	60 seconds
3A. Stepup (racked) (page 74)	3	12 per leg	None
3B. Single-Leg Romanian Deadlift (page 100)	3	12 per leg	60 seconds
4A. Lunge (racked) (page 64)	3	12 per leg	None
4B. Side Lunge (racked) (page 65)	3	12 per leg	60 seconds
5A. Turkish Getup (page 132)	2	12 per side	None
5B. Double Windmill (page 135)	2	12 per side	None
5C. Crunch (page 51)	2	12	45 seconds

WEEK 1 *(cont.)*

Workouts 2 and 4

EXERCISES	SETS	REPS	REST
1A. Around-the-Legs Pass (warmup) (page 95)	1	30 seconds	None
1B. Standing Twist (warmup) (page 73)	1	30 seconds	None
1C. Halo (warmup) (page 116)	1	30 seconds	None
2A. Chest Press (page 48)	4	10	None
2B. Chest Fly (page 50)	4	10	None
2C. Pullover (page 83)	4	10	< 60 seconds
3A. 45-Degree Two-Arm Row (page 99)	4	10	None
3B. Yates Row (page 99)	4	10	< 60 seconds
4A. Two-Hand Shoulder Press (page 119)	4	10	None
4B. Iron Cross (page 117)	4	10	None
4C. Seesaw Press (page 119)	4	10	< 60 seconds
5A. Biceps Curl (page 46)	4	10	None
5B. Lying Triceps Extension (page 80)	4	10	< 60 seconds

WEEK 2

Workouts 1 and 3

EXERCISES	SETS	REPS	REST
1A. Standing Twist (warmup) (page 73)	1	30 seconds	None
1B. Around-the-Body Pass (warmup) (page 94)	1	30 seconds	None
1C. Halo (warmup) (page 116)	1	30 seconds	None
1D. Single-Arm Swing (warmup) (page 106)	1	12 per arm (using 2 kettlebells)	30 seconds
2A. Double Clean (page 90)	4	10	None
2B. Front Squat (racked) (page 53)	4	10	60 seconds
3A. Stepup (racked) (page 74)	4	10 per leg	None
3B. Single-Leg Romanian Deadlift (page 100)	4	10 per leg	60 seconds
4A. Lunge (racked) (page 64)	4	10 per leg	None
4B. Side Lunge (racked) (page 65)	4	10 per leg	60 seconds
5A. Turkish Getup (page 132)	3	12 per side	None
5B. Double Windmill (page 135)	3	12 per side	None
5C. Crunch (page 51)	3	12	45 seconds

WEEK 2 *(cont.)*

Workouts 2 and 4

EXERCISES	SETS	REPS	REST
1A. Around-the-Legs Pass (warmup) (page 95)	1	30 seconds	None
1B. Standing Twist (warmup) (page 73)	1	30 seconds	None
1C. Halo (warmup) (page 116)	1	30 seconds	None
2A. Chest Press (page 48)	4	10	None
2B. Chest Fly (page 50)	4	10	None
2C. Pullover (page 83)	4	10	< 60 seconds
3A. 45-Degree Two-Arm Row (page 99)	4	10	None
3B. Yates Row (page 99)	4	10	< 60 seconds
4A. Two-Hand Shoulder Press (page 119)	4	10	None
4B. Iron Cross (page 117)	4	10	None
4C. Seesaw Press (page 119)	4	10	< 60 seconds
5A. Biceps Curl (page 46)	4	10	None
5B. Lying Triceps Extension (page 80)	4	10	< 60 seconds

WEEK 3

Workouts 1 and 3

EXERCISES	SETS	REPS	REST
1A. Standing Twist (warmup) (page 73)	1	30 seconds	None
1B. Around-the-Body Pass (warmup) (page 94)	1	30 seconds	None
1C. Halo (warmup) (page 116)	1	30 seconds	None
1D. Single-Arm Swing (warmup) (page 106)	2	10 per arm (using 2 kettlebells)	30 seconds
2. Front Squat (racked) (page 53)	2	12	< 75 seconds
3. Romanian Deadlift (page 100)	2	12	< 75 seconds
4. Wide-Stance Goblet Squat (page 127)	2	12	< 75 seconds
5A. Straight-Leg Deadlift (page 59)	3	12	None
5B. Single-Leg Romanian Deadlift (page 100)	3	12 per leg	< 45 seconds
6A. Lunge (racked) (page 64)	3	12 per leg	None
6B. Side Lunge (racked) (page 65)	3	12 per leg	< 45 seconds
7A. Turkish Getup (page 132)	3	12 per side	None
7B. Double Windmill (page 135)	3	12 per side	None
7C. Crunch (page 51)	3	12	30 seconds

WEEK 3 (cont.)

Workouts 2 and 4

EXERCISES	SETS	REPS	REST
1A. Around-the-Legs Pass (warmup) (page 95)	1	As many as possible in 30 seconds	None
1B. Standing Twist (warmup) (page 73)	1	As many as possible in 30 seconds	None
1C. Halo (warmup) (page 116)	1	As many as possible in 30 seconds	None
1D. Pushups (page 114)	1	12	
2. Chest Press (page 48)	2	12	< 75 seconds
3. 45-Degree Two-Arm Row (page 99)	2	12	< 75 seconds
4. Two-Hand Shoulder Press (page 119)	2	12	< 75 seconds
5A. Chest Fly (page 50)	3	12	None
5B. Pullover (page 83)	3	12	< 45 seconds
6. Renegade Row and Burpee (page 131)	3	12	< 45 seconds
7A. Seesaw Press (page 119)	3	12	None
7B. Iron Cross (page 117)	3	12	< 45 seconds
8. Biceps Curl (page 46)	2	12	< 75 seconds
9. Lying Triceps Extension (page 80)	2	12	< 75 seconds

WEEK 4

Workouts 1 and 3

EXERCISES	SETS	REPS	REST
1A. Standing Twist (warmup) (page 73)	1	30 seconds	None
1B. Around-the-Body Pass (warmup) (page 94)	1	30 seconds	None
1C. Halo (warmup) (page 116)	1	30 seconds	None
1D. Single-Arm Swing (warmup) (page 106)	2	10 per arm (using 2 kettlebells)	30 seconds
2. Front Squat (racked) (page 53)	3	10	< 75 seconds
3. Romanian Deadlift (page 100)	3	10	< 75 seconds
4. Wide-Stance Goblet Squat (page 127)	3	10	< 75 seconds
5A. Straight-Leg Deadlift (page 59)	4	12	None
5B. Single-Leg Romanian Deadlift (page 100)	4	12 per leg	< 45 seconds
6A. Lunge (racked) (page 64)	4	12 per leg	None
6B. Side Lunge (racked) (page 65)	4	12 per leg	< 45 seconds
7A. Turkish Getup (page 132)	4	12 per side	None
7B. Double Windmill (page 135)	4	12 per side	None
7C. Crunch (page 51)	4	12	30 seconds

WEEK 4 *(cont.)*

Workouts 2 and 4

EXERCISES	SETS	REPS	REST
1A. Around-the-Legs Pass (warmup) (page 95)	1	30 seconds	None
1B. Standing Twist (warmup) (page 73)	1	30 seconds	None
1C. Halo (warmup) (page 116)	1	30 seconds	None
1D. Pushup (page 114)	1	12	
2. Chest Press (page 48)	3	10	< 75 seconds
3. 45-Degree Two-Arm Row (page 99)	3	10	< 75 seconds
4. Two-Hand Shoulder Press (page 119)	3	10	< 75 seconds
5A. Chest Fly (page 50)	4	12	None
5B. Pullover (page 83)	4	12	< 45 seconds
6. Renegade Row and Burpee (page 131)	4	12	< 45 seconds
7A. Seesaw Press (page 119)	4	12	None
7B. Iron Cross (page 117)	4	12	< 45 seconds
8. Biceps Curl (page 46)	3	10	< 75 seconds
9. Lying Triceps Extension (page 80)	3	10	< 75 seconds

Sandbag Muscle Builder

Although exercise equipment made from iron is the traditional choice for building muscle, you can still pack on plenty of it using the right sandbag routine. (If possible, try to have several different sizes of sandbags available.) This 4-week program designed by master sandbag instructor Josh Gonzalez combines 3 days of unique exercise programming for maximum muscle size.

RULES TO REMEMBER

● Use this plan for 4 weeks, 3 days a week, taking at least 48 hours to recover between workouts.

● Each day, you'll be performing a series of supersets—exercises performed back-to-back with no rest between. Perform the required number of repetitions of the first exercise (the A exercise) at a 2/0/2 tempo: Take 2 seconds to raise the weight and 2 seconds to lower it, with no pause in between.

● Perform the second exercise (the B exercise) for the required amount of time. Lower the sandbag as slowly as possible, trying to bring that muscle to failure. After performing both exercises, rest for 60 to 90 seconds, and repeat.

● Always perform a comprehensive warmup before and a cooldown after each workout.

ABOUT THE EXPERT

Josh Gonzalez, NASM-CPT, has 17 years of experience in the fitness industry, specializing in sports performance, speed development, and unconventional fitness training. Josh is a master instructor for the National Academy of Sports Medicine, a master instructor for DVRT Ultimate Sandbag Training, and the owner of Athletic Performance of Texas in Longview, Tyler, and Austin, Texas.

WEEK 1

Workout 1

EXERCISES	SETS	REPS OR TIME	REST
1A. High Pull (page 112)	3	12	None
1B. Deadlift (page 56)	3	60 seconds	60–90 seconds
2A. Rotating High Pull (page 154)	3	12 on right side only	None
2B. Vertical Single-Leg Row (page 181)	3	60 seconds on right side only	60–90 seconds
3A. Rotating High Pull (page 154)	3	12 on left side only	None
3B. Vertical Single-Leg Row (page 181)	3	60 seconds on left side only	60–90 seconds
4A. Zercher Squat (page 145)	3	12	None
4B. Good Morning Front Squat (page 169)	3	60 seconds	60–90 seconds

Workout 2

EXERCISES	SETS	REPS OR TIME	REST
1A. Clean (page 140)	3	12	None
1B. Lateral Drag (page 182)	3	60 seconds	60–90 seconds
2A. Lunge (page 64)	3	12 on right side only	None
2B. Kneeling Shoulder-to-Shoulder Press (page 179)	3	60 seconds	60–90 seconds
3A. Lunge (page 64)	3	12 on left side only	None
3B. Kneeling Shoulder-to-Shoulder Press (page 179)	3	60 seconds	60–90 seconds
4A. Zercher Squat (page 145)	3	12	None
4B. Shoveling (page 152)	3	60 seconds	60–90 seconds

Workout 3

EXERCISES	SETS	REPS OR TIME	REST
1A. Clean and Press (page 158)	3	12	None
1B. Zercher Squat and Press (page 145)	3	60 seconds	60–90 seconds
2A. Side Lunge Clean (page 175)	3	12	None
2B. Alternating Rotating Lunge (page 157)	3	60 seconds	60–90 seconds
3A. Rotating Clean Lunge Press (page 149)	3	12	None
3B. High Pull (page 112)	3	60 seconds	60–90 seconds

WEEK 2

Workout 1

EXERCISES	SETS	REPS	REST
1A. High Pull (page 112)	3	10	None
1B. Deadlift (page 56)	3	10	60–90 seconds
2A. Rotating High Pull (page 154)	3	10 on right side only	None
2B. Vertical Single-Leg Row (page 181)	3	10 on right side only	60–90 seconds
3A. Rotating High Pull (page 154)	3	10 on left side only	None
3B. Vertical Single-Leg Row (page 181)	3	10 on left side only	60–90 seconds
4A. Zercher Squat (page 145)	3	10	None
4B. Good Morning Front Squat (page 169)	3	10	60–90 seconds

Workout 2

EXERCISES	SETS	REPS	REST
1A. Clean (page 140)	3	10	None
1B. Lateral Drag (page 182)	3	10	60–90 seconds
2A. Lunge (page 64)	3	10 on right side only	None
2B. Kneeling Shoulder-to-Shoulder Press (page 179)	3	10	60–90 seconds
3A. Lunge (page 64)	3	10 on left side only	None
3B. Kneeling Shoulder-to-Shoulder Press (page 179)	3	10	60–90 seconds
4A. Zercher Squat (page 145)	3	10	None
4B. Shoveling (page 152)	3	10	60–90 seconds

Workout 3

EXERCISES	SETS	REPS	REST
1A. Clean and Press (page 158)	3	10	None
1B. Zercher Squat and Press (page 145)	3	10	60–90 seconds
2A. Side Lunge Clean (page 175)	3	10	None
2B. Alternating Rotating Lunge (page 157)	3	10	60–90 seconds
3A. Rotating Clean Lunge Press (page 149)	3	10	None
3B. High Pull (page 112)	3	10	60–90 seconds

WEEK 3

Workout 1

EXERCISES	SETS	REPS	REST
1A. High Pull (page 112)	3	8	None
1B. Deadlift (page 56)	3	8	60–90 seconds
2A. Rotating High Pull (page 154)	3	8 on right side only	None
2B. Vertical Single-Leg Row (page 181)	3	8 on right side only	60–90 seconds
3A. Rotating High Pull (page 154)	3	8 on left side only	None
3B. Vertical Single-Leg Row (page 181)	3	8 on left side only	60–90 seconds
4A. Zercher Squat (page 145)	3	8	None
4B. Good Morning Front Squat (page 169)	3	8	60–90 seconds

Workout 2

EXERCISES	SETS	REPS	REST
1A. Clean (page 140)	3	8	None
1B. Lateral Drag (page 182)	3	8	60–90 seconds
2A. Lunge (page 64)	3	8 on right side only	None
2B. Kneeling Shoulder-to-Shoulder Press (page 179)	3	8	60–90 seconds
3A. Lunge (page 64)	3	8 on left side only	None
3B. Kneeling Shoulder-to-Shoulder Press (page 179)	3	8	60–90 seconds
4A. Zercher Squat (page 145)	3	8	None
4B. Shoveling (page 152)	3	8	60–90 seconds

Workout 3

EXERCISES	SETS	REPS	REST
1A. Clean and Press (page 158)	3	8	None
1B. Zercher Squat and Press (page 145)	3	8	60–90 seconds
2A. Side Lunge Clean (page 175)	3	8	None
2B. Alternating Rotating Lunge (page 157)	3	8	60–90 seconds
3A. Rotating Clean Lunge Press (page 149)	3	8	None
3B. High Pull (page 112)	3	8	60–90 seconds

WEEK 4

Workout 1

EXERCISES	SETS	REPS	REST
1A. High Pull (page 112)	3	6	None
1B. Deadlift (page 56)	3	6	60–90 seconds
2A. Rotating High Pull (page 154)	3	6 on right side only	None
2B. Vertical Single-Leg Row (page 181)	3	6 on right side only	60–90 seconds
3A. Rotating High Pull (page 154)	3	6 on left side only	None
3B. Vertical Single-Leg Row (page 181)	3	6 on left side only	60–90 seconds
4A. Zercher Squat (page 145)	3	6	None
4B. Good Morning Front Squat (page 169)	3	6	60–90 seconds

Workout 2

EXERCISES	SETS	REPS	REST
1A. Clean (page 140)	3	6	None
1B. Lateral Drag (page 182)	3	6	60–90 seconds
2A. Lunge (page 64)	3	6 on right side only	None
2B. Kneeling Shoulder-to-Shoulder Press (page 179)	3	6	60–90 seconds
3A. Lunge (page 64)	3	6 on left side only	None
3B. Kneeling Shoulder-to-Shoulder Press (page 179)	3	6	60–90 seconds
4A. Zercher Squat (page 145)	3	6	None
4B. Shoveling (page 152)	3	6	60–90 seconds

Workout 3

EXERCISES	SETS	REPS	REST
1A. Clean and Press (page 158)	3	6	None
1B. Zercher Squat and Press (page 145)	3	6	60–90 seconds
2A. Side Lunge Clean (page 175)	3	6	None
2B. Alternating Rotating Lunge (page 157)	3	6	60–90 seconds
3A. Rotating Clean Lunge Press (page 149)	3	6	None
3B. High Pull (page 112)	3	6	60–90 seconds

Dumbbell Performance Booster

For advice on building a physique capable of handling any sport, we chose a trainer who has worked with athletes from high school to the Olympics, plus professional football, baseball, basketball, and hockey players. NASM master instructor Tony Ambler-Wright designed the following progressive month-long training cycle so that each workout affects your neuromuscular system differently every time you exercise. This tactic is critical for the development of the ultimate athlete.

"An athlete's body needs to respond under every possible circumstance and be able to perform at its highest level, which is why a program that's never the same twice can be the best approach," says Ambler-Wright. "Best of all, because each workout places a unique demand on the body and incorporates a variety of training intensities, directions of motion, and speeds of movement, this program will prevent boredom, minimize overtraining, maximize recovery, and most importantly, optimize results."

RULES TO REMEMBER

● Use this plan for 4 weeks, 3 days a week, taking at least 48 hours to recover between workouts.

● Workout 1 is a moderately intense superset program that improves strength endurance. Perform the exercises marked with an asterisk at a controlled tempo, going slower on the negative or lowering portion of the lift.

● Workout 2 is a lower-intensity program for movement efficiency, stability, and endurance. Perform this conditioning circuit of nine moves at a slow and controlled tempo, especially the negative portion of each lift.

● Workout 3 is a high-intensity superset program that improves power endurance. Exercises marked with an asterisk should be performed explosively as quickly as possible. Exercises without the asterisk should be performed at a moderate to high intensity.

ABOUT THE EXPERT

Tony Ambler-Wright, MS, LMT, CSCS, is a training systems and program development coordinator for Atlanta-based sports science company Fusionetics.

WEEK 1

Workout 1

EXERCISES	SETS	REPS	REST
*__1A.__ Bottom-Half Getup (page 165)	2	4 per side	None
__1B.__ Neutral-Grip Deadlift (page 57)	2	12	None
*__1C.__ Single-Leg Romanian Deadlift (page 58)	2	8 per side	None

Rest for 60–90 seconds and repeat 1A–1C for the recommended number of sets.

__2A.__ Chest Press (page 48)	2	12	None
*__2B.__ Pushup Drag (page 67)	2	8	None
__2C.__ Yates Row (page 99)	2	12	None
*__2D.__ Cross-Bench Pullover (page 83)	2	8	None

Rest for 60–90 seconds and repeat 2A–2D for the recommended number of sets.

__3A.__ Goblet Squat (page 126)	2	12	None
*__3B.__ Bulgarian Isometric Squat (page 55)	2	8 per side	None
__3C.__ Seated (or Kneeling) Lateral Raise (page 61)	2	12	None
*__3D.__ Reverse Woodchop (page 79)	2	8 per side	None

Rest for 60–90 seconds and repeat 3A–3D for the recommended number of sets.

*Perform the negative slowly.

WEEK 1 *(cont.)*

Workout 2

EXERCISES	SETS	REPS	REST
T-Pushup (page 67)	2	12	None
Reverse Crunch (page 70)	2	12	None
Stepup (page 74)	2	12 per side	None
Renegade Row (page 130)	2	12	None
Side Plank (page 72)	2	12 (hold 5 seconds per rep)	None
Side Lunge (page 65)	2	12	None
Single-Arm Shoulder Press (page 84)	2	12 per side	None
Single-Leg Woodchop (page 79)	2	12 per side	None
Crossover Stepup (page 75)	2	12 per side	None

Rest for 60–90 seconds and repeat the circuit.

Workout 3

EXERCISES	SETS	REPS	REST
1A. Windmill (page 134)	2	4 per side	None
***1B.** Snatch (page 86)	2	8 per side	None
Rest 2 minutes and repeat 1A–1B for the recommended number of sets.			
2A. Floor Press (page 49)	2	8	None
***2B.** Alternating Chest Press (page 49)	2	20	None
2C. Walking Lunge (page 65)	2	8 per leg	None
***2D.** Double-Arm Swing (page 108)	2	10	None
Rest for 2 minutes and repeat 2A–2D for the recommended number of sets.			
3A. Two-Arm Row (page 76)	2	8	None
***3B.** Lawnmower Pull (page 76)	2	10 per side	None
3C. Front Squat (page 53)	2	8	None
***3D.** Jump Squat (page 55)	2	10	None
Rest for 2 minutes and repeat 3A–3D for the recommended number of sets.			

Perform the negative slowly.

WEEK 2

Workout 1

EXERCISES	SETS	REPS	REST
*1A. Bottom-Half Getup (page 165)	3	4 per side	None
1B. Neutral-Grip Deadlift (page 57)	3	12	None
*1C. Single-Leg Romanian Deadlift (page 58)	3	8 per side	None

Rest for 60–90 seconds and repeat 1A–1C for the recommended number of sets.

2A. Alternating Chest Press (page 49)	3	12	None
*2B. Pushup Drag (page 67)	3	8	None
2C. Yates Row (page 99)	3	12	None
*2D. Cross-Bench Pullover (page 83)	3	8	None

Rest for 60–90 seconds and repeat 2A–2D for the recommended number of sets.

3A. Goblet Squat (page 126)	3	12	None
*3B. Bulgarian Isometric Squat (page 55)	3	8 per side	None
3C. Seated (or Kneeling) Lateral Raise (page 61)	3	12	None
*3D. Reverse Woodchop (page 79)	3	8 per side	None

Rest for 60–90 seconds and repeat 3A–3D for the recommended number of sets.

*Perform the negative slowly.

Workout 2

EXERCISES	SETS	REPS	REST
T-Pushup (page 67)	2	16	None
Reverse Crunch (page 70)	2	16	None
Stepup (page 74)	2	16	None
Renegade Row (page 130)	2	16	None
Side Plank (page 72)	2	16 (hold 5 seconds per rep)	None
Side Lunge (page 65)	2	16	None
Single-Arm Shoulder Press (page 84)	2	16 per side	None
Single-Leg Woodchop (page 79)	2	16 per side	None
Crossover Stepup (page 75)	2	16 per side	None

Rest for 60–90 seconds and repeat the circuit.

WEEK 2 *(cont.)*

Workout 3

EXERCISES	SETS	REPS	REST
1A. Windmill (page 134)	3	4 per side	None
***1B.** Snatch (page 86)	3	8 per side	None
Rest 2 minutes and repeat 1A–1B for the recommended number of sets.			
2A. Floor Press (page 49)	3	8	None
***2B.** Alternating Chest Press (page 49)	3	20	None
2C. Walking Lunge (page 65)	3	8 per leg	None
***2D.** Double-Arm Swing (page 108)	3	10	None
Rest for 2 minutes and repeat 2A–2D for the recommended number of sets.			
3A. Two-Arm Row (page 76)	3	8	None
***3B.** Lawnmower Pull (page 76)	3	10 per side	None
3C. Front Squat (page 53)	3	8	None
***3D.** Jump Squat (page 55)	3	10	None
Rest for 2 minutes and repeat 3A–3D for the recommended number of sets.			

Perform the negative slowly.

WEEK 3

Workout 1

EXERCISES	SETS	REPS	REST
*1A. Bottom-Half Getup (page 165)	3	3 per side	None
1B. Neutral-Grip Deadlift (page 57)	3	10	None
*1C. Single-Leg Romanian Deadlift (page 58)	3	10 per side	None
Rest for 60–90 seconds and repeat 1A–1C for the recommended number of sets.			
2A. Chest Press (page 48)	3	10	None
*2B. Pushup Drag (page 67)	3	10	None
2C. Yates Row (page 99)	3	10	None
*2D. Cross-Bench Pullover (page 83)	3	10	None
Rest for 60–90 seconds and repeat 2A–2D for the recommended number of sets.			
3A. Goblet Squat (page 126)	3	10	None
*3B. Bulgarian Isometric Squat (page 55)	3	10 per side	None
3C. Seated (or Kneeling) Lateral Raise (page 61)	3	10	None
*3D. Reverse Woodchop (page 79)	3	10 per side	None
Rest for 60–90 seconds and repeat 3A–3D for the recommended number of sets.			

*Perform the negative slowly.

WEEK 3 *(cont.)*

Workout 2

EXERCISES	SETS	REPS	REST
T-Pushup (page 67)	3	12	None
Reverse Crunch (page 70)	3	12	None
Stepup (page 74)	3	12 per side	None
Renegade Row (page 130)	3	12	None
Side Plank (page 72)	3	12 (hold 5 seconds per rep)	None
Side Lunge (page 65)	3	12	None
Single-Arm Shoulder Press (page 84)	3	12 per side	None
Single-Leg Woodchop (page 79)	3	12 per side	None
Crossover Stepup (page 75)	3	12 per side	None

Rest for 60–90 seconds and repeat the circuit twice more.

Workout 3

EXERCISES	SETS	REPS	REST
1A. Windmill (page 134)	3	3 per side	None
***1B.** Snatch (page 86)	3	6 per side	None
Rest 2 minutes and repeat 1A–1B for the recommended number of sets.			
2A. Floor Press (page 49)	3	6	None
***2B.** Alternating Chest Press (page 49)	3	20	None
2C. Walking Lunge (page 65)	3	6 per leg	None
***2D.** Double-Arm Swing (page 108)	3	10	None
Rest for 2 minutes and repeat 2A–2D for the recommended number of sets.			
3A. Two-Arm Row (page 76)	3	6	None
***3B.** Lawnmower Pull (page 76)	3	10 per side	None
3C. Front Squat (page 53)	3	6	None
***3D.** Jump Squat (page 55)	3	10	None
Rest for 2 minutes and repeat 3A–3D for the recommended number of sets.			

*Perform explosively and quickly.

WEEK 4

Workout 1

EXERCISES	SETS	REPS	REST
*1A. Bottom-Half Getup (page 165)	3	2 per side	None
1B. Neutral-Grip Deadlift (page 57)	3	8	None
*1C. Single-Leg Romanian Deadlift (page 58)	3	12 per side	None
Rest for 60–90 seconds and repeat 1A–1C for the recommended number of sets.			
2A. Alternating Chest Press (page 49)	3	8	None
*2B. Pushup Drag (page 67)	3	12	None
2C. Yates Row (page 99)	3	8	None
*2D. Cross-Bench Pullover (page 83)	3	12	None
Rest for 60–90 seconds and repeat 2A–2D for the recommended number of sets.			
3A. Goblet Squat (page 126)	3	8	None
*3B. Bulgarian Isometric Squat (page 55)	3	12 per side	None
3C. Seated (or Kneeling) Lateral Raise (page 61)	3	8	None
*3D. Reverse Woodchop (page 79)	3	12 per side	None
Rest for 60–90 seconds and repeat 3A–3D for the recommended number of sets.			

*Perform the negative slowly.

Workout 2

EXERCISES	SETS	REPS	REST
T-Pushup (page 67)	3	16	None
Reverse Crunch (page 70)	3	16	None
Stepup (page 74)	3	16 per side	None
Renegade Row (page 130)	3	16	None
Side Plank (page 72)	3	16 (hold 5 seconds per rep)	None
Side Lunge (page 65)	3	16	None
Single-Arm Shoulder Press (page 84)	3	16 per side	None
Single-Leg Woodchop (page 79)	3	16 per side	None
Crossover Stepup (page 75)	3	16 per side	None

Rest for 60–90 seconds and repeat the circuit twice more.

WEEK 4 *(cont.)*

Workout 3

EXERCISES	SETS	REPS	REST
1A. Windmill (page 134)	4	3 per side	None
***1B.** Snatch (page 86)	4	6 per side	None
Rest 2 minutes and repeat 1A–1B for the recommended number of sets.			
2A. Floor Press (page 49)	4	6	None
***2B.** Alternating Chest Press (page 49)	4	20	None
2C. Walking Lunge (page 65)	4	6 per leg	None
***2D.** Double-Arm Swing (page 108)	4	10	None
Rest for 2 minutes and repeat 2A–2D for the recommended number of sets.			
3A. Two-Arm Row (page 76)	4	6	None
***3B.** Lawnmower Pull (page 76)	4	10 per side	None
3C. Front Squat (page 53)	4	6	None
***3D.** Jump Squat (page 55)	4	10	None
Rest for 2 minutes and repeat 3A–3D for the recommended number of sets.			

Perform explosively and quickly.

Kettlebell Performance Booster

Personal trainer Chip Huss follows the philosophy that athletes need to be strong in awkward, unpredictable positions, so he trains people for sports in an unorthodox way. His 6-week program uses exercises that build dynamic flexibility, functional stability, and a tremendous amount of mind-body awareness and control. The exercises in this routine will leave you with explosive strength, flexible hips, a solid core, and super-strong shoulders, so you'll move with more efficiency and athletic precision.

RULES TO REMEMBER

- Depending on your rate of progress, use this program for at least 6 weeks or as long as 8 weeks, taking 48 hours to recover between workouts.

- Make sure you do the exercises in the order they're listed and select the proper weight. You want to be able to maintain proper form, but you should need the 60-second rest between exercises. If you don't feel like you need the rest time, add more weight.

- Always perform a warmup before and a cooldown after each workout.

ABOUT THE EXPERT

Chip Huss, MS, NASM-CPT, CSCS, specializes in performance enhancement and injury prevention. Huss previously worked alongside chiropractors for the Denver Broncos, is a master instructor for the National Academy of Sports Medicine, and works with Olympians, professional boxers, mixed martial arts fighters, tactical athletes, first responders, and postrehab patients at Champion Breed Boxing and Mixed Martial Arts. The Colorado-based trainer is also the head athletic performance trainer for Don Beebe's House of Speed, a training camp for improving athletic speed.

WEEKS 1–6

Workout 1

EXERCISES	SETS	REPS	REST
Halo (page 116)	1	5 per side	60 seconds
45-Degree Two-Arm Row (page 99)	1	10	60 seconds
Double Clean (page 90)	1	8	60 seconds
Double High Pull (page 113)	1	8	60 seconds
Reverse Lunge (page 122)	1	8 per side	60 seconds
Renegade Row with Burpee (page 131)	1	8	60 seconds
Double Windmill (page 135)	1	8	60 seconds

Rest for 5 minutes, then repeat the circuit twice more, for a total of 3 circuits.

Workout 2

EXERCISES	SETS	REPS	REST
Turkish Getup (page 132)	1	10 per side	60 seconds
Sots Press (page 121)	1	6 per arm	60 seconds
Single-Leg Romanian Deadlift (page 100)	1	6 per leg	60 seconds
Alternating Single-Arm Swing (page 107)	1	10 per arm	60 seconds
Bottom-Up Shoulder Press (page 119)	1	10 per arm	60 seconds
Wide-Stance Goblet Squat (page 127)	1	10	60 seconds
One-Arm High Pull (page 113)	1	10 per arm	60 seconds

Rest for 4 minutes, then repeat the circuit twice, for a total of 3 circuits.

Workout 3

EXERCISES	SETS	REPS	REST
Figure-Eight (page 96)	1	10	60 seconds
Pushup Drag (page 115)	1	10	60 seconds
Two-Hand Snatch (page 111)	1	10	60 seconds
Seesaw Press (page 119)	1	10	60 seconds
Pistol Squat (alternating legs) (page 128)	1	5 per leg	60 seconds
Single-Arm Push Press (page 120)	1	5 per arm	60 seconds
Death Crawl (page 115)	1	10	60 seconds

Rest for 5 minutes, then repeat the circuit twice, for a total of 3 circuits.

Sandbag Performance Booster

Performance coach Marty Miller knows that whether you're a weekend warrior, an exercise junkie, or a competitive athlete at any level, it's essential to condition your muscles with movements that teach your body to work explosively and generate more power with less fatigue. Miller also knows that sandbag training can take your performance to that next level, which is why he designed a routine that simultaneously improves strength, stamina, and stability. His 4-week program starts by introducing basic, total-body sandbag movements, then shifts into more complex sandbag movements, while also increasing the intensity and volume—and decreasing the rest intervals between exercises—as you progress from week to week.

RULES TO REMEMBER

- Use this plan for 4 weeks, 3 days a week, taking at least 48 hours off between workouts to give your body time to recover.

- Perform this workout as a circuit, moving from one exercise to the next after one set and resting for the given time.

- Always perform a comprehensive warmup before and cooldown after each workout.

ABOUT THE EXPERT

Marty Miller, DHSc, ATC, CSCS, is a National Academy of Sports Medicine master instructor and director of fitness at Mizner Country Club in Delray Beach, Florida, with more than 20 years of experience in sports medicine, performance enhancement, and injury prevention. He has worked with both the Montreal Expos and the New York Yankees.

WEEK 1

Workout 1

EXERCISES	SETS	REPS OR DISTANCE	REST
Bear Hug Squat (page 139)	2	12–20	60 seconds
Drag (page 160)	2	40 feet	60 seconds
Bottom-Half Getup (page 165)	2	12	60 seconds
Offset Farmer's Walk (page 163)	2	40 feet per side	60 seconds
Clean (page 140)	2	12	60 seconds
Shouldering (page 142)	2	12	60 seconds
Single-Arm Swing (page 176)	2	12 per side	60 seconds
Biceps Curl (page 46)	2	12	60 seconds
Overhead Triceps Extension (page 82)	2	12	60 seconds

Complete 1 set of each exercise, then repeat the circuit.

WEEK 1 *(cont.)*

Workout 2

EXERCISES	SETS	REPS OR DISTANCE	REST
Wide-Stance Bear Hug Squat (page 139)	2	12–20	60 seconds
Drag (page 160)	2	50 feet	60 seconds
Bottom-Half Getup (page 165)	2	12–15	60 seconds
Overhead Farmer's Walk (page 163)	2	80 feet	60 seconds
Good Morning Front Squat (page 169)	2	12	60 seconds
Clean and Press (page 158)	2	12	60 seconds
Pushup (page 170)	2	12	60 seconds
Standard Crunch (page 147)	2	12	60 seconds
Shoveling (page 152)	2	12	60 seconds

Complete 1 set of each exercise, then repeat the circuit.

Workout 3

EXERCISES	SETS	REPS OR DISTANCE	REST
Lunge (page 64)	2	12–20 per leg	60 seconds
Bear Hug Farmer's Walk (page 163)	2	80 feet	60 seconds
Offset Drag (page 161)	2	40 feet per side	60 seconds
Clean and Press (page 158)	2	12–15	60 seconds
Side Crunch Hip Thrust (page 165)	2	12 per side	60 seconds
Single-Leg Woodchop (page 79)	2	12 each side	60 seconds
Lateral Drag (page 182)	2	12	60 seconds
Rotating Deadlift (page 150)	2	12	60 seconds
Rotating Hang Pull (page 154)	2	12	60 seconds

Complete 1 set of each exercise, then repeat the circuit.

WEEK 2

Workout 1

EXERCISES	SETS	REPS OR DISTANCE	REST
Bear Hug Squat (page 139)	3	12–20	45 seconds
Drag (page 160)	3	80 feet	45 seconds
Bottom-Half Getup (page 165)	3	12	45 seconds
Offset Farmer's Walk (page 163)	3	50 feet per side	45 seconds
Clean (page 140)	3	12	45 seconds
Shouldering (page 142)	3	12	45 seconds
Single-Arm Swing (page 176)	3	12 per side	45 seconds
Biceps Curl (page 46)	3	12–15	45 seconds
Overhead Triceps Extension (page 82)	3	12–15	45 seconds

Complete 1 set of each exercise, then repeat the circuit two more times.

Workout 2

EXERCISES	SETS	REPS OR DISTANCE	REST
Wide-Stance Bear Hug Squat (page 139)	3	12–20	45 seconds
Drag (page 160)	3	50–75 feet	45 seconds
Bottom-Half Getup (page 165)	3	12–15	45 seconds
Overhead Farmer's Walk (page 163)	3	80–100 feet	45 seconds
Good Morning Front Squat (page 169)	3	12–15	45 seconds
Clean and Press (page 158)	3	12–15	45 seconds
Pushup (page 170)	3	12–15	45 seconds
Standard Crunch (page 147)	3	12–15	45 seconds
Shoveling (page 152)	3	12–15	45 seconds

Complete 1 set of each exercise, then repeat the circuit two more times.

Workout 3

EXERCISES	SETS	REPS OR DISTANCE	REST
Reverse Lunge (page 172)	3	12–15	45 seconds
One-Arm Overhead Farmer's Walk (page 163)	3	30 feet each side	45 seconds
Staggered Stance Clean and Press (page 158)	3	12	45 seconds
Turkish Getup (page 166)	3	5 each side	45 seconds
Single-Leg Woodchop (page 79)	3	12 each side	45 seconds
Alternating Rotating Deadlift (page 151)	3	16	45 seconds
Rotating High Pull (page 154)	3	12	45 seconds
Pushup (page 170)	3	12–20	45 seconds

Complete 1 set of each exercise, then repeat the circuit two more times.

WEEK 3

Workout 1

EXERCISES	SETS	REPS OR DISTANCE	REST
Clean and Lunge (page 173)	3	15	30 seconds
Around-the-World (page 155)	3	15 per side	30 seconds
Turkish Getup (page 166)	3	6 per side	30 seconds
Overhead Farmer's Walk (page 163)	3	100 feet	30 seconds
Staggered Stance Clean and Press (page 158)	3	15	30 seconds
One-Arm Shouldering (page 143)	3	8 per side	30 seconds
Overhead Raise Long-Arm Crunch (page 147)	3	15	30 seconds
Biceps Curl (page 46)	3	15	30 seconds
Overhead Triceps Extension (page 82)	3	15	30 seconds

Complete 1 set of each exercise, then repeat the circuit two more times.

Workout 2

EXERCISES	SETS	REPS OR DISTANCE	REST
Wide-Stance Bear Hug Squat (page 139)	3	15	30 seconds
One-Arm Drag (page 161)	3	50 feet per arm	30 seconds
Bear Hug Good Morning (page 169)	3	15	30 seconds
Rotating High Pull (page 154)	3	15	30 seconds
Side Lunge Shouldering (page 143)	3	15 per side	30 seconds
Chest Press (page 48)	3	15	30 seconds
Side-to-Side Pickup (page 171)	3	8 per side	30 seconds
Rotating Lunge Clean (page 157)	3	8 per leg	30 seconds
Single-Leg Row (page 180)	3	8 per side	30 seconds

Complete 1 set of each exercise, then repeat the circuit two more times.

Workout 3

EXERCISES	SETS	REPS OR DISTANCE	REST
Clean and Lunge (page 173)	3	8 per leg	30 seconds
One-Arm Overhead Farmer's Walk (page 163)	3	100 feet	30 seconds
Rotating Snatch (page 144)	3	8 per side	30 seconds
Turkish Getup (page 166)	3	8 per side	30 seconds
Zercher Squat and Press (page 145)	3	15	30 seconds
Pushup (page 170)	3	15	30 seconds
Push Press (page 68)	3	15	30 seconds
Kneeling Shoulder-to-Shoulder Press (page 179)	3	8 per side	30 seconds

Complete 1 set of each exercise, then repeat the circuit two more times.

WEEK 4

Workout 1

EXERCISES	SETS	REPS OR DISTANCE	REST
Clean and Lunge (page 173)	3	20	30 seconds
Around-the-World (page 155)	3	20 per side	30 seconds
Turkish Getup (page 166)	3	10 per side	30 seconds
One-Arm Overhead Farmer's Walk (page 163)	3	75 feet per arm	30 seconds
Rotating Snatch (page 144)	3	10 per side	30 seconds
Side Lunge Shouldering (page 143)	3	10 per side	30 seconds
Long-Arm Crunch (page 146)	3	20	30 seconds
Biceps Curl (page 46)	3	20	30 seconds
Overhead Triceps Extension (page 82)	3	20	30 seconds

Complete 1 set of each exercise, then repeat the circuit two more times.

Workout 2

EXERCISES	SETS	REPS OR DISTANCE	REST
Wide-Stance Bear Hug Squat (page 139)	3	20	30 seconds
One-Arm Drag (page 161)	3	75 feet per arm	30 seconds
Single-Leg Good Morning (page 169)	3	10 per leg	30 seconds
Rotating Clean and Press (page 149)	3	10 per side	30 seconds
One-Arm Shouldering (page 143)	3	10 per side	30 seconds
Chest Press (page 48)	3	20	30 seconds
Side-to-Side Pickup (page 171)	3	10 per side	30 seconds
Side Lunge Deadlift (page 175)	3	10 per side	30 seconds
*Side-to-Side Pickup (page 171)	3	10 per side	30 seconds

Complete 1 set of each exercise, then repeat the circuit two more times.

*Repeat Side-to-Side Pickup.

Workout 3

EXERCISES	SETS	REPS OR DISTANCE	REST
Staggered Stance Clean and Press (page 158)	3	20	30 seconds
One-Arm Overhead Farmer's Walk (page 163)	3	125 feet	30 seconds
Zercher Squat and Press (page 145)	3	20	30 seconds
Chest Press (page 48)	3	20	30 seconds
Turkish Getup (page 166)	3	10 per side	30 seconds
Wiper (page 177)	3	20	30 seconds
Rotating Snatch (page 144)	3	10 per side	30 seconds
Side Lunge/Shoulder-to-Shoulder Press (page 179)	3	10 per side	30 seconds

Complete 1 set of each exercise, then repeat the circuit two more times.

INDEX

Boldface page references indicate photographs. Underscored references indicate boxed text.

A

Abdominal muscles, 32
Abduction, 6
Adduction, 6
Afterburn, 222
Almonds, 39
Alternating Chest Press, 49, **49**
Alternating Rotating Deadlift, 151, **151**
Alternating Rotating Lunge Clean, 157, **157**
Alternating Single-Arm Swing, 107, **107**
Arc Press, 179, **179**
Around-the-Body Pass, 94–95, **94–95**
Around-the-Legs Pass, 95, **95**
Around-the-World, 155, **155**

B

Banana, 39, 40
Bear Hug, 138, **138**
Bear Hug Farmer's Walk, 163, **163**
Bear Hug Good Morning, 169, **169**
Bear Hug Squat, 139, **139**
Beginner 3-Day Workout, 195
Bent-Over Row
    dumbbell, 77, **77**
    kettlebell, 98–99, **98–99**
    Neutral-Grip, 181, **181**
    Staggered Stance, 181, **181**
Bent Press, 101, **101**
Biceps brachii, 29–30
Biceps Curl, **46**, 46–47
Bilateral training, 10–11
Bird Dog, 104, **104**
Blueberries, <u>95</u>
Body type, 10
Bottom-Half Getup, 165, **165**
Bottom-Up Shoulder Press, 119, **119**
Bowflex, 21
Breakfast
    ideal, 40
    minimeal before, 39–40
Bulgarian Isometric Squat, 55, **55**

C

Calf Raise
    Seated, 63, **63**
    Single-Leg, 63, **63**
Calories
    burned by
        digestion, 36, 37
        drinking chilled water, 41
        jumping rope between exercises, <u>162</u>
        sandbag exercises, <u>141</u>
        unilateral training, 11
    determining number needed, 36
    dividing into seven meals, 36
Calves, 29
Carbohydrates, 38–39
    benefits of, 39
    calories per gram, 39
    daily amount needed, 38–39
    low- and high-glycemic, 39
    in pre- and postworkout meal, <u>37</u>
    sources, 39
Cardiovascular health, kettlebell exercises for, 15
Casein protein, 41
Catabolic state, 39, 41
Cheese, <u>37</u>, 41
Chest Fly, 50, **50**
    Incline, 50, **50**
Chest (pectorals) muscles, 28
Chest Press, 48–49, **48–49**
    Alternating, 49, **49**
    Incline, 49, **49**
Circuit training, <u>190</u>
Clean
    kettlebell, 90–91, **90–91**
    sandbag, **140**, 140–41
Clean and Lunge, 173, **173**
Clean and Press
    dumbbell, 52, **52**
    kettlebell, 92–93, **92–93**
    sandbag, 158, **158**
Compound exercises, 204, 213, 238
Connective tissue, increasing elasticity with warmup, <u>194</u>
Core exercises
    dumbbell exercises, 197
    kettlebell exercises, 198
    sandbag exercises, 199
Cortisol, 40

Cross-Bench Pullover, 83, **83**
Crossover Stepup, 75, **75**
Crunch, 51, **51**
    Double, 70, **70**
    Long-Arm, 51, **51**, 146–47,
        146–47
    Overhead Raise Long-Arm,
        147, **147**
    Reverse, 70, **70**
    Side Crunch Hip Thrust, 165,
        165
    Standard, 147, **147**

D

Dead Clean, 91, **91**
Deadlift
    Alternating Rotating, 151, **151**
    Double, 97, **97**
    dumbbell, 56–57, **56–57**
    kettlebell, 97, **97**
    Neutral-Grip, 57, **57**
    Romanian, 58, **58**, 100, **100**
    Rotating, 150–51, **150–51**
    Single-Leg Romanian, 58, **58**,
        100, **100**
    Single-Leg Straight-Leg, 59, **59**
    Straight-Leg, 59, **59**
    Sumo, 57, **57**
Death Crawl, 115, **115**
Dehydration, 40
Deltoids, 30
Diet, 35–41
Digestion, calories burned by, 36,
    37
Double-Arm Swing, 108–9,
    108–9
Double Clean, 90, **90**
Double Clean and Press, 93, **93**
Double Crunch, 70, **70**
Double Deadlift, 97, **97**
Double High Pull, 113, **113**
Double Swing, 109, **109**
Double Windmill, 135, **135**
Drag, 160–61, **160–61**
    Lateral, 182, **182**
    Offset, 161, **161**

One-Arm, 161, **161**
    Pushup, 67, **67**, 115, **115**
Drinking as you exercise, 40–41
Dumbbell(s). *See also* Dumbbell
    exercises; Dumbbell
    workouts
    advantages of, 11–12
        ease of mastery, 12
        muscle specificity, 12
        strength building, 12
    choosing, 20–21
    history of, 11
    1-Week Test Drive routine,
        188–89
    types
        fixed-weight, 20
        plate-loaded adjustable,
            20–21
        selectorized adjustable, 20,
            21
    where to purchase, 21
Dumbbell exercises, 45–87
    Alternating Chest Press, 49,
        49
    Bent-Over Row, 77, **77**
    Biceps Curl, **46**, 46–47
    Bulgarian Isometric Squat, 55,
        55
    Chest Fly, 50, **50**
    Chest Press, 48–49, **48–49**
    Clean and Press, 52, **52**
    Cross-Bench Pullover, 83, **83**
    Crossover Stepup, 75, **75**
    Crunch, 51, **51**
    Deadlift, 56–57, **56–57**
    Double Crunch, 70, **70**
    exercise cheat sheet, 197
    Floor Press, 49, **49**
    Front Squat, 53, **53**
    Hang Pull, 85, **85**
    Incline Chest Fly, 50, **50**
    Incline Chest Press, 49, **49**
    Incline Hammer Curl, 47, **47**
    Jump Squat, 55, **55**
    Kneeling Twist, 71, **71**
    Lateral Raise, 60–61, **60–61**
    Lateral T-Raise, 61, **61**
    Lawnmower Pull, 77, **77**

Long-Arm Crunch, 51, **51**
Lunge, 64–65, **64–65**
Lying Triceps Extension, 80,
    80
Neutral-Grip Deadlift, 57, **57**
Overhead Triceps Extension,
    82, **82**
Prone Hammer Curl, 47, **47**
Pullover, 83, **83**
Push Press, 68, **68**
Pushup, 66–67, **66–67**
Pushup Drag, 67, **67**
Rear Lateral Raise, 62, **62**
Reverse Crunch, 70, **70**
Romanian Deadlift, 58, **58**
Russian Twist, 71, **71**
sandbag exercises compared,
    141
Seated Calf Raise, 63, **63**
Seated (or Kneeling) Lateral
    Raise, 61, **61**
Shrug, 69, **69**
Side Lunge, 65, **65**
Side Plank, 72, **72**
Single-Arm Lateral Raise, 61,
    61
Single-Arm Shoulder Press,
    84, **84**
Single-Arm Triceps Kickback,
    81, **81**
Single-Leg Calf Raise, 63, **63**
Single-Leg Romanian
    Deadlift, 58, **58**
Single-Leg Row, 76, **76**
Single-Leg Straight-Leg
    Deadlift, 59, **59**
Single-Leg Woodchop, 79, **79**
Snatch, 86–87, **86–87**
Squat, 54–55, **54–55**
Standing Shoulder Press, 84,
    84
Standing Twist, 73, **73**
Stepup, 74–75, **74–75**
Straight-Leg Deadlift, 59, **59**
substituting for kettlebell or
    sandbag exercises, 87
Sumo Deadlift, 57, **57**
Tate Press, 79, **79**

T-Pushup, 67, **67**
Two-Arm Row, 76, **76**
Two-Arm Triceps Kickback,
    81, **81**
Walking Lunge, 65, **65**
Woodchop, 78–79, **78–79**
Zottman Curl, 47, **47**
Dumbbell workouts
    Dumbbell Fat Blaster, 213–21
        Week 1, 214–15
        Week 2, 216–17
        Week 3, 218–19
        Week 4, 220–21
    Dumbbell Muscle Builder,
        229–37
        Week 1, 230–31
        Week 2, 232–33
        Week 3, 234–35
        Week 4, 236–37
    Dumbbell Performance
        Booster, 256–68
        Week 1, 257–59
        Week 2, 260–62
        Week 3, 263–65
        Week 4, 266–68

E

Eating, 35–41
    before bed, 41
    macronutrients, 37–39
    meals as reward, 41
    minimeal before breakfast,
        39–40
    pre- and postworkout eating
        plan, 37
    for target body weight, 36
    whey protein shake recipes,
        39–40
Eggs, 40
Elephant, parable of blind men
        and, 3–4, **4**
EPOC, 222
Erector spinae, 32
Excess post-exercise oxygen
        consumption (EPOC),
        222

Exercise(s). *See also* Workouts
    bilateral and unilateral, 10–11
    drinking as you exercise,
        40–41
    dumbbell, 45–87
        Alternating Chest Press, 49,
            49
        Bent-Over Row, 77, **77**
        Biceps Curl, **46**, 46–47
        Bulgarian Isometric Squat,
            55, **55**
        Chest Fly, 50, **50**
        Chest Press, 48–49, **48–49**
        Clean and Press, 52, **52**
        Cross-Bench Pullover, 83,
            83
        Crossover Stepup, 75, **75**
        Crunch, 51, **51**
        Deadlift, 56–57, **56–57**
        Double Crunch, 70, **70**
        exercise cheat sheet, 197
        Floor Press, 49, **49**
        Front Squat, 53, **53**
        Hang Pull, 85, **85**
        Incline Chest Fly, 50, **50**
        Incline Chest Press, 49, **49**
        Incline Hammer Curl, 47,
            47
        Jump Squat, 55, **55**
        Kneeling Twist, 71, **71**
        Lateral Raise, 60–61, **60–61**
        Lateral T-Raise, 61, **61**
        Lawnmower Pull, 77, **77**
        Long-Arm Crunch, 51, **51**
        Lunge, 64–65, **64–65**
        Lying Triceps Extension,
            80, **80**
        Neutral-Grip Deadlift, 57,
            57
        Overhead Triceps
            Extension, 82, **82**
        Prone Hammer Curl, 47, **47**
        Pullover, 83, **83**
        Push Press, 68, **68**
        Pushup, 66–67, **66–67**
        Pushup Drag, 67, **67**
        Rear Lateral Raise, 62, **62**
        Reverse Crunch, 70, **70**

        Romanian Deadlift, 58, **58**
        Russian Twist, 71, **71**
        Seated Calf Raise, 63, **63**
        Seated (or Kneeling)
            Lateral Raise, 61, **61**
        Shrug, 69, **69**
        Side Lunge, 65, **65**
        Side Plank, 72, **72**
        Single-Arm Lateral Raise,
            61, **61**
        Single-Arm Shoulder Press,
            84, **84**
        Single-Arm Triceps
            Kickback, 81, **81**
        Single-Leg Calf Raise, 63,
            63
        Single-Leg Romanian
            Deadlift, 58, **58**
        Single-Leg Row, 76, **76**
        Single-Leg Straight-Leg
            Deadlift, 59, **59**
        Single-Leg Woodchop, 79,
            79
        Snatch, 86–87, **86–87**
        Squat, 54–55, **54–55**
        Standing Shoulder Press,
            84, **84**
        Standing Twist, 73, **73**
        Stepup, 74–75, **74–75**
        Straight-Leg Deadlift, 59, **59**
        Sumo Deadlift, 57, **57**
        Tate Press, 79, **79**
        T-Pushup, 67, **67**
        Two-Arm Row, 76, **76**
        Two-Arm Triceps
            Kickback, 81, **81**
        Walking Lunge, 65, **65**
        Woodchop, 78–79, **78–79**
        Zottman Curl, 47, **47**
    kettlebell, 89–135
        Alternating Single-Arm
            Swing, 107, **107**
        Around-the-Body Pass,
            94–95, **94–95**
        Around-the-Legs Pass, 95,
            95
        Bent-Over Row, 98–99,
            98–99

Exercise(s)

kettlebell *(cont.)*

Bent Press, 101, **101**

Bird Dog, 104, **104**

Bottom-Up Shoulder Press, 119, **119**

Clean, 90–91, **90–91**

Clean and Press, 92–93, **92–93**

Dead Clean, 91, **91**

Deadlift, 97, **97**

Death Crawl, 115, **115**

Double-Arm Swing, 108–9, **108–9**

Double Clean, 90, **90**

Double Clean and Press, 93, **93**

Double Deadlift, 97, **97**

Double High Pull, 113, **113**

Double Swing, 109, **109**

Double Windmill, 135, **135**

Farmer's Walk, 102–3, **102–3**

Figure-Eight, 96, **96**

45-Degree Two-Arm Row, 99, **99**

Goblet Lunge, 123, **123**

Goblet Squat, 126–27, **126–27**

Half-Getup, 133, **133**

Half-Turn Swing, 109, **109**

Halo, 116, **116**

Hang Clean, 91, **91**

High Pull, 112–13, **112–13**

Hip Flexor Rainbow, 105, **105**

Hip Flexor Stretch, 105, **105**

Hip Hinge and Stretches, 104–5, **104–5**

Iron Cross, 117, **117**

One-Arm High Pull, 113, **113**

Overhead Farmer's Walk, 103, **103**

Overhead Lunge, 123, **123**

Pistol Squat, 128–29, **128–29**

Pushup, 114–15, **114–15**

Pushup Drag, 115, **115**

Pushup-Position Plank, 105, **105**

Rack Walk, 103, **103**

Renegade Row, 130–31, **130–31**

Renegade Row and Burpee, 131, **131**

Reverse Lunge, 122–23, **122–23**

Romanian Deadlift, 100, **100**

safety during, 14–15, 93

saving your forearms during, 91

Seesaw Press, 119, **119**

Shoulder Press, 118–19, **118–19**

Single-Arm Push Press, 120, **120**

Single-Arm Swing, 106–7, **106–7**, 107

Single-Leg Romanian Deadlift, 100, **100**

Single-Leg Row, 99, **99**

Six-Point Zenith, 105, **105**

Snatch, 110–11, **110–11**

Sots, 121, **121**

substituting for dumbbell exercises, 135

Suitcase Carry, 103, **103**

Tactical Lunge, 124, **124–25**

Thruster, 127, **127**

Turkish Getup, 132–33, **132–33**

Two-Arm Push Press, 120, **120**

Two-Hand Shoulder Press, 119, **119**

Two-Hand Snatch, 111, **111**

Walking Swing, 109, **109**

Wall Drill, 104, **104**

Wide-Stance Goblet Squat, 127, **127**

Windmill, 134–35, **134–35**

Yates Row, 99, **99**

muscles adapting to, 10

in planes of motion, 6

sandbag, 137–83

Alternating Rotating Deadlift, 151, **151**

Alternating Rotating Lunge Clean, 157, **157**

Arc Press, 179, **179**

Around-the-World, 155, **155**

Bear Hug, 138, **138**

Bear Hug Farmer's Walk, 163, **163**

Bear Hug Good Morning, 169, **169**

Bear Hug Squat, 139, **139**

Bottom-Half Getup, 165, **165**

Clean, **140**, 140–41

Clean and Lunge, 173, **173**

Clean and Press, 158, **158**

Drag, 160–61, **160–61**

Farmer's Walk, 162–63, **162–63**

Getup, 164–65, **164–65**

Good Morning, 168–69, **168–69**

Good Morning Squat, 169, **169**

Grip Curl, 159, **159**

Kneeling Shoulder-to-Shoulder Press, 179, **179**

Lateral Drag, 182, **182**

Long-Arm Crunch, 146–47, **146–47**

Neutral-Grip Bent-Over-Row, 181, **181**

Offset Drag, 161, **161**

Offset Farmer's Walk, 163, **163**

One-Arm Drag, 161, **161**

One-Arm Overhead Farmer's Walk, 163, **163**

One-Arm Shouldering, 143, **143**

Overhead Farmer's Walk, 163, **163**

Overhead Raise Long-Arm Crunch, 147, **147**

Pushup, 170, **170**

Reverse Lunge, 172–73, **172–73**

Rotating Clean, 148–49, **148–49**
Rotating Clean and Press, 149, **149**
Rotating Clean Lunge Press, 149, **149**
Rotating Deadlift, 150–51, **150–51**
Rotating Hang Pull, 154, **154**
Rotating Lunge, 156–57, **156–57**
Rotating Snatch, 144, **144**
Rotational Reverse Lunge, 173, **173**
Shouldering, 142–43, **142–43**
Shoulder Leg Threading, 165, **165**
Shoulder-to-Shoulder Press, 178–79, **178–79**
Shoveling, 152, **152**
Shucking, 153, **153**
Side Crunch Hip Thrust, 165, **165**
Side Lunge, 174–75, **174–75**
Side Lunge Clean, 175, **175**
Side Lunge Shouldering, 143, **143**
Side Lunge/Shoulder-to-Shoulder Press, 179, **179**
Side-to-Side Pickup, 171, **171**
Single-Arm Swing, 176, **176**
Single-Leg Good Morning, 169, **169**
Single-Leg Row, 180–81, **180–81**
Snatch, 144, **144**
Staggered Stance Bent-Over Row, 181, **181**
Staggered Stance Clean and Press, 158, **158**
Staggered Stance Shoulder-to-Shoulder Press, 179, **179**
Standard Crunch, 147, **147**
Swing, 176, **176**
Turkish Getup, 166–67, **166–67**

Vertical Single-Leg Row, 181, **181**
Wide-Stance Bear Hug Squat, 139, **139**
Zercher Squat, 145, **145**
Zercher Squat and Press, 145, **145**
Exercise machines, 10
Exercise type cheat sheet, 197–99
    dumbbell exercises, 197
    kettlebell exercises, 198
    sandbag exercises, 199
External obliques, 32

F

Failure, stopping one rep short of, <u>194</u>
Farmer's Walk
    Bear Hug, 163, **163**
    kettlebell, 102–3, **102–3**
    Offset, 163, **163**
    One-Arm Overhead, 163, **163**
    Overhead, 103, **103**, 163, **163**
    sandbag, 162–63, **162–63**
Fat
    burning with
        drinking chilled water, 36
        increase meal frequency, 36
        kettlebell exercises, 36
    calories per gram, 38
    daily amount needed, 38
    health benefits of, 38
    healthy fats, 38
    reduction with
        blueberries, <u>95</u>
        eating before bed, 41
    sources, 38
Fat blaster workouts
    Dumbbell Fat Blaster, 213–21
    Kettlebell Fat Blaster, 222–26
    Sandbag Fat Blaster, 227–28
Fatty acids, omega-3 and omega-6, 38
Figure-Eight, 96, **96**
Floor Press, 49, **49**
Foam rolling, 227

Food. *See* Eating; *specific foods*
Forearm muscles, 30
Form, <u>46</u>, <u>93</u>
45-Degree Two-Arm Row, 99, **99**
Frontal plane, 5–6
Front Squat, 53, **53**

G

Gastrocnemius, 29
Gear. *See* Tools
Getup, 164–65, **164–65**
    Bottom-Half, 165, **165**
    Half-Getup, 133, **133**
    Turkish, 132–33, **132–33**
Glucose, <u>37</u>
Gluteals, 31–32
Glycogen, <u>37</u>
Goblet Lunge, 123, **123**
Goblet Squat, 126–27, **126–27**
Good Morning, 168–69, **168–69**
    Bear Hug, 169, **169**
    Single-Leg, 169, **169**
Good Morning Squat, 169, **169**
Grip Curl, 159, **159**
Grip strength increase with sandbag exercises, 16
Growth hormone, boost with Kettlebell Swings, <u>111</u>

H

Half-Getup, 133, **133**
Half-Turn Swing, 109, **109**
Halo, 116, **116**
Halteres, 11
Hammer Curl
    Incline, 47, **47**
    Prone, 47, **47**
Hamstrings, 30
Hang Clean, 91, **91**
Hang Pull, 85, **85**
Heart rate, elevation with sandbag exercises, <u>141</u>
    unilateral training, 11
High-intensity interval training (HIIT), 222

High Pull, 112–13, **112–13**
    Double, 113, **113**
    One-Arm, 113, **113**
HIIT, 222
Hip Flexor Rainbow, 105, **105**
Hip flexors, 33
Hip Flexor Stretch, 105, **105**
Hip Hinge and Stretches, 104–5, **104–5**
    Bird Dog, 104, **104**
    Hip Flexor Rainbow, 105, **105**
    Hip Flexor Stretch, 105, **105**
    Pushup-Position Plank, 105, **105**
    Six-Point Zenith, 105, **105**
    Wall Drill, 104, **104**
Horizontal loading, 229
Horizontal plane, 5–6
Hunger, 37, 41
Hydration, 40–41

I

Iliacus, 33
Imbalances, 4, 7, 11, 15
Incline Chest Fly, 50, **50**
Incline Chest Press, 49, **49**
Incline Hammer Curl, 47, **47**
Insulin, <u>37</u>
Insulin sensitivity, 36, <u>95</u>
Intermediate 4-Day Workout, 196
Intermediate 3-Day Workout, 195
Internal obliques, 32
Intervals
    high-intensity interval training (HIIT), 222
    Tabata, 204, 206, 222–26
Iron Cross, 117, **117**

J

Jogging, as warmup, <u>194</u>
Jumping jacks, as warmup, <u>194</u>

Jumping rope
    between exercises, <u>162</u>
    as warmup, <u>194</u>
Jump Squat, 55, **55**

K

Kettlebell(s), 5. *See also* Kettlebell exercises; Kettlebell workouts
    advantages of, 5, 12–15
        fat burning, 15
        the handle, 13
        hybrid lifts, 13
        metabolism boost, 15
        nonsymmetrical weight distribution, 13
        safety of, 14–15
        strengthening the mind-muscle connection, 14
        use of posterior muscles, 14
    history of, 13
    1-Week Test Drive routine, 189
    picking, <u>22</u>, 22–23
    sizes, 21
    where to purchase, <u>22</u>
Kettlebell exercises, 89–135
    Alternating Single-Arm Swing, 107, **107**
    Around-the-Body Pass, 94–95, **94–95**
    Around-the-Legs Pass, 95, **95**
    Bent-Over Row, 98–99, **98–99**
    Bent Press, 101, **101**
    Bottom-Up Shoulder Press, 119, **119**
    Clean, 90–91, **90–91**
    Clean and Press, 92–93, **92–93**
    Dead Clean, 91, **91**
    Deadlift, 97, **97**
    Death Crawl, 115, **115**
    Double-Arm Swing, 108–9, **108–9**
    Double Clean, 90, **90**
    Double Clean and Press, 93, **93**
    Double Deadlift, 97, **97**

    Double High Pull, 113, **113**
    Double Swing, 109, **109**
    Double Windmill, 135, **135**
    exercise cheat sheet, 198
    Farmer's Walk, 102–3, **102–3**
    Figure-Eight, 96, **96**
    45-Degree Two-Arm Row, 99, **99**
    Goblet Lunge, 123, **123**
    Goblet Squat, 126–27, **126–27**
    Half-Getup, 133, **133**
    Half-Turn Swing, 109, **109**
    Halo, 116, **116**
    Hang Clean, 91, **91**
    High Pull, 112–13, **112–13**
    Hip Hinge and Stretches, 104–5, **104–5**
        Bird Dog, 104, **104**
        Hip Flexor Rainbow, 105, **105**
        Hip Flexor Stretch, 105, **105**
        Pushup-Position Plank, 105, **105**
        Six-Point Zenith, 105, **105**
        Wall Drill, 104, **104**
    Iron Cross, 117, **117**
    One-Arm High Pull, 113, **113**
    Overhead Farmer's Walk, 103, **103**
    Overhead Lunge, 123, **123**
    Pistol Squat, 128–29, **128–29**
    Pushup, 114–15, **114–15**
    Pushup Drag, 115, **115**
    Rack Walk, 103, **103**
    Renegade Row, 130–31, **130–31**
    Renegade Row and Burpee, 131, **131**
    Reverse Lunge, 122–23, **122–23**
    Romanian Deadlift, 100, **100**
    safety during, 14–15, <u>93</u>
    saving your forearms during, <u>91</u>
    Seesaw Press, 119, **119**
    Shoulder Press, 118–19, **118–19**
    Single-Arm Push Press, 120, **120**

Single-Arm Swing, 106–7, **106–7**, <u>107</u>
Single-Leg Romanian Deadlift, 100, **100**
Single-Leg Row, 99, **99**
Snatch, 110–11, **110–11**
Sots, 121, **121**
substituting for dumbbell exercises, 135
Suitcase Carry, 103, **103**
Tactical Lunge, 124, **124–25**
Thruster, 127, **127**
Turkish Getup, 132–33, **132–33**
Two-Arm Push Press, 120, **120**
Two-Hand Shoulder Press, 119, **119**
Two-Hand Snatch, 111, **111**
Walking Swing, 109, **109**
Wide-Stance Goblet Squat, 127, **127**
Windmill, 134–35, **134–35**
Yates Row, 99, **99**
The Kettlebell Shredder, 204–7
 4-week plan, 205
 Workout 1: Simple Strength, 205
 Workout 2: Killer Cardio, 206
 Workout 3: Sweat Cyclone, 206
 Workout 4: Tonic Recharge, 207
 Workout 5: Mobility, 207
Kettlebell workouts
 Kettlebell Fat Blaster, 222–26
  Week 1, 223
  Week 2, 224
  Week 3, 225
  Week 4, 226
 Kettlebell Muscle Builder, 238–46
  Week 1, 239–40
  Week 2, 241–42
  Week 3, 243–44
  Week 4, 245–46
 Kettlebell Performance Booster, 269–71

The Kettlebell Shredder, 204–7
 4-week plan, 205
 Workout 1: Simple Strength, 205
 Workout 2: Killer Cardio, 206
 Workout 3: Sweat Cyclone, 206
 Workout 4: Tonic Recharge, 207
 Workout 5: Mobility, 207
Kneeling Shoulder-to-Shoulder Press, 179, **179**
Kneeling Twist, 71, **71**

L

Lateral Drag, 182, **182**
Lateral Raise, 60–61, **60–61**
Lateral T-Raise, 61, **61**
Latissimus dorsi, 29
Lawnmower Pull, 77, **77**
Lingo, <u>190</u>
Long-Arm Crunch
 dumbbell, 51, **51**
 Overhead Raise, 147, **147**
 sandbag, 146–47, **146–47**
Lower back muscles, 32
Lower body pull exercises
 dumbbell exercises, 197
 kettlebell exercises, 198
 sandbag exercises, 199
Lower body push exercises
 dumbbell exercises, 197
 kettlebell exercises, 198
 sandbag exercises, 199
Lunge
 Alternating Rotating Lunge Clean, 157, **157**
 Clean and Lunge, 173, **173**
 dumbbell, 64–65, **64–65**
 Goblet, 123, **123**
 Overhead, 123, **123**
 Reverse, 122–23, **122–23**, 172–73, **172–73**
 Rotating, 156–57, **156–57**
 Rotating Clean Lunge Press, 149, **149**
 Rotational Reverse, 173, **173**
 Side, 65, **65**, 174–75, **174–75**
 Side Lunge Clean, 175, **175**
 Side Lunge Shouldering, 143, **143**
 Side Lunge/Shoulder-to-Shoulder Press, 179, **179**
 Tactical, 124, **124–25**
 Walking, 65, **65**
 as warmup exercise, <u>125</u>
Lying Triceps Extension, 80, **80**

M

Macronutrients
 carbohydrate, 38–39
 fat, 38
 protein, 37–38
Mass, workouts for
 Dumbbell Muscle Builder, 229–37
 Kettlebell Muscle Builder, 238–46
 Sandbag Muscle Builder, 247–55
Meals
 frequency of, 36
 minimeal before breakfast, 39–40
 pre- and postworkout eating plan, <u>37</u>
 as reward, <u>41</u>
Metabolism increase with
 drinking chilled water, 41
 kettlebell exercises, 15
 protein prior to training session, <u>69</u>, <u>151</u>
Mind-muscle connection, strengthening with kettlebells, 14
Mirror muscles, 7
Motion, planes of, 5–6
Movement mastery, kickstarters for
 The Kettlebell Shredder, 204–7
 The Sandstorm, 208–12

Muscle Builder workouts
  Dumbbell Muscle Builder,
    229–37
  Kettlebell Muscle Builder,
    238–46
  Sandbag Muscle Builder,
    247–55
Muscle building basics, 201
Muscles, 27–33
  adapting to an exercise, 10
  anatomical location, **31**
  breakdown in catabolic state,
    39, 41
  building symmetrical, 10
  fast twitch fibers, 15
  imbalances, 4, 7, 11, 15
  mirror, 7
  proprioceptive, 10, 13
  that help pull, 29–30
    biceps brachii, 29–30
    forearm (wrist extensors
      and wrist flexors), 30
    hamstrings, 30
    latissimus dorsi, 29
    rhomboids, 29
    trapezius, 29
  that help push, 28–29
    calves, 29
    chest (pectorals), 28
    quadriceps, 28–29
    triceps brachii, 28
  that help swing, 32–33
    abdominals, 32
    hip flexors, 33
    lower back, 32
  that push and pull, 30–32
    deltoids, 30
    gluteals, 31–32
  warming up, 194

N

Neutral-Grip Bent-Over-Row,
  181, **181**
Neutral-Grip Deadlift, 57, **57**
Nutrition, 35–41

O

Obliques, 32
Offset Drag, 161, **161**
Offset Farmer's Walk, 163, **163**
Omega-3 and omega-6 fatty
  acids, 38
One-Arm Drag, 161, **161**
One-Arm High Pull, 113, **113**
One-Arm Overhead Farmer's
  Walk, 163, **163**
One-Arm Shouldering, 143, **143**
1-rep rule, 194
1-Week Test Drives, 187–90
  dumbbell, 188–89
  kettlebell, 189
  sandbag, 190
Overhead Farmer's Walk, 103,
  103, 163, **163**
Overhead Lunge, 123, **123**
Overhead Raise Long-Arm
  Crunch, 147, **147**
Overhead Triceps Extension, 82,
  82

P

Pectoral muscles, 28
Performance, workouts for
  Dumbbell Performance
    Booster, 256–68
  Kettlebell Performance
    Booster, 269–71
  Sandbag Performance Booster,
    272–81
Pistol Squat, 128–29, **128–29**
Planes of motion, 5–6
Posterior chain, 14
Posture, 7
PowerBlock, 21
Prone Hammer Curl, 47, **47**
Proprioceptive muscles, 10, 13
Protein, 37–38
  before bed, 41
  calories per gram, 38
  daily amount needed, 37
  in pre- and postworkout meal,
    37
  prior to training session for
    metabolism boost, 69, 151
  sources, 38
  whey protein shake, 39–40
Protein shake, 37, 39–40, 41
Psoas major, 33
Pull, muscles that help, 29–30
  biceps brachii, 29–30
  deltoids, 30
  forearm (wrist extensors and
    wrist flexors), 30
  gluteals, 31–32
  hamstrings, 30
  latissimus dorsi, 29
  rhomboids, 29
  trapezius, 29
Pull exercises, 4
  lower body
    dumbbell exercises, 197
    kettlebell exercises, 198
    sandbag exercises, 199
  upper body
    dumbbell exercises, 197
    kettlebell exercises, 198
    sandbag exercises, 199
Pullover, 83, **83**
  Cross-Bench, 83, **83**
Push, muscles that help, 28–29
  calves, 29
  chest (pectorals), 28
  deltoids, 30
  gluteals, 31–32
  quadriceps, 28–29
  triceps brachii, 28
Push exercises
  lower body
    dumbbell exercises, 197
    kettlebell exercises, 198
    sandbag exercises, 199
  overloading workout with, 4
  upper body
    dumbbell exercises, 197
    kettlebell exercises, 198
    sandbag exercises, 199
Push Press, 68, **68**

Pushup
    dumbbell, 66–67, **66–67**
    kettlebell, 114–15, **114–15**
    sandbag, 170, **170**
Pushup Drag
    dumbbell, 67, **67**
    kettlebell, 115, **115**
Pushup-Position Plank, 105,
    105

Q

Quadriceps, 28–29

R

Rack Walk, 103, **103**
Rear Lateral Raise, 62, **62**
Rectus abdominis, 32
Rectus femoris, 28
Renegade Row, 130–31, **130–31**
Renegade Row and Burpee, 131,
    131
Repetition (rep)
    defined, 190
    number of reps, 201
    1-rep rule, 194
Resistance training
    jumping rope between
        exercises, 162
    warming up before, 190
Rest (rest interval)
    defined, 190
    jumping rope between
        exercises, 162
    length and number of
        workouts per week, 201
Return policy, for sandbags, 23,
    25
Reverse Crunch, 70, **70**
Reverse Lunge
    kettlebell, 122–23, **122–23**
    sandbag, 172–73, **172–73**
Rhomboids, 29
Rogue Fitness bags, 25

Romanian Deadlift
    dumbbell, 58, **58**
    kettlebell, 100, **100**
    Single-Leg, 58, **58**, 100, **100**
Rotating Clean, 148–49, **148–49**
Rotating Clean and Press, 149,
    149
Rotating Clean Lunge Press, 149,
    149
Rotating Deadlift, 150–51,
    150–51
Rotating Hang Pull, 154, **154**
Rotating Lunge, 156–57, **156–57**
Rotating Snatch, 144, **144**
Rotational motion, 6
Rotational Reverse Lunge, 173,
    173
Routines. *See* Workouts
Russian Twist, 71, **71**

S

Safety during kettlebell
        exercises, 14–15, 93
Sagittal plane, 5–6
Sand, 17, 23
Sandbag. *See also* Sandbag
        exercises; Sandbag
        workouts
    advantages of, 5, 16–17
        functional strength
            development, 17
        grip strength increase, 16
        inexpensive, 16
        shifting center of mass, 16
        travel friendly, 17
        unconventional nature of,
            17
    making your own gear, 24
    1-Week Test Drive routine, 190
    origins of, 15–16
    picking perfect, 23, 25
    where to purchase, 25
Sandbag exercises, 137–83
    adding difficulty to workout,
        208

Alternating Rotating Deadlift,
    151, **151**
Alternating Rotating Lunge
    Clean, 157, **157**
Arc Press, 179, **179**
Around-the-World, 155, **155**
Bear Hug, 138, **138**
Bear Hug Farmer's Walk, 163,
    163
Bear Hug Good Morning, 169,
    169
Bear Hug Squat, 139, **139**
Bottom-Half Getup, 165, **165**
Clean, 140, 140–41
Clean and Lunge, 173, **173**
Clean and Press, 158, **158**
Drag, 160–61, **160–61**
dumbbell exercises compared,
    141
exercise cheat sheet, 199
Farmer's Walk, 162–63,
    162–63
Getup, 164–65, **164–65**
Good Morning, 168–69,
    168–69
Good Morning Squat, 169, **169**
Grip Curl, 159, **159**
Kneeling Shoulder-to-
    Shoulder Press, 179, **179**
Lateral Drag, 182, **182**
Long-Arm Crunch, 146–47,
    146–47
Neutral-Grip Bent-Over-Row,
    181, **181**
Offset Drag, 161, **161**
Offset Farmer's Walk, 163, **163**
One-Arm Drag, 161, **161**
One-Arm Overhead Farmer's
    Walk, 163, **163**
One-Arm Shouldering, 143,
    143
Overhead Farmer's Walk, 163,
    163
Overhead Raise Long-Arm
    Crunch, 147, **147**
Pushup, 170, **170**
Reverse Lunge, 172–73, **172–73**

Sandbag exercises *(cont.)*
  Rotating Clean, 148–49, **148–49**
  Rotating Clean and Press, 149, **149**
  Rotating Clean Lunge Press, 149, **149**
  Rotating Deadlift, 150–51, **150–51**
  Rotating Hang Pull, 154, **154**
  Rotating Lunge, 156–57, **156–57**
  Rotating Snatch, 144, **144**
  Rotational Reverse Lunge, 173, **173**
  Shouldering, 142–43, **142–43**
  Shoulder Leg Threading, 165, **165**
  Shoulder-to-Shoulder Press, 178–79, **178–79**
  Shoveling, 152, **152**
  Shucking, 153, **153**
  Side Crunch Hip Thrust, 165, **165**
  Side Lunge, 174–75, **174–75**
  Side Lunge Clean, 175, **175**
  Side Lunge Shouldering, 143, **143**
  Side Lunge/Shoulder-to-Shoulder Press, 179, **179**
  Side-to-Side Pickup, 171, **171**
  Single-Arm Swing, 176, **176**
  Single-Leg Good Morning, 169, **169**
  Single-Leg Row, 180–81, **180–81**
  Snatch, 144, **144**
  Staggered Stance Bent-Over-Row, 181, **181**
  Staggered Stance Clean and Press, 158, **158**
  Staggered Stance Shoulder-to-Shoulder Press, 179, **179**
  Standard Crunch, 147, **147**
  substituting for dumbbell or kettlebell exercises, 183
  Swing, 176, **176**
  Turkish Getup, 166–67, **166–67**
  Vertical Single-Leg Row, 181, **181**
  Wide-Stance Bear Hug Squat, 139, **139**
  Zercher Squat, 145, **145**
  Zercher Squat and Press, 145, **145**
Sandbag workouts
  Sandbag Fat Blaster, 227–28
  Sandbag Muscle Builder, 247–55
    Week 1, 248–49
    Week 2, 250–51
    Week 3, 252–53
    Week 4, 254–55
  Sandbag Performance Booster, 272–81
    Week 1, 273–75
    Week 2, 276–77
    Week 3, 278–79
    Week 4, 280–81
  The Sandstorm, 208–12
    adding difficulty to workout, 208
    Week 1, 209
    Week 2, 210
    Week 3, 211
    Week 4, 212
  The Sandstorm (workout), 208–12
    adding difficulty to workout, 208
    Week 1, 209
    Week 2, 210
    Week 3, 211
    Week 4, 212
Seated Calf Raise, 63, **63**
Seated (or Kneeling) Lateral Raise, 61, **61**
Seesaw Press, 119, **119**
Self-myofascial release (SMR), 227
Sets
  defined, 190
  number of sets, 201
Shake, whey protein, 39–40
Shoes, flat-soled workout, 93
Shouldering, 142–43, **142–43**
Shoulder Leg Threading, 165, **165**
Shoulder Press, 118–19, **118–19**
  Bottom-Up, 119, **119**
  Kneeling Shoulder-to-Shoulder Press, 179, **179**
  Shoulder-to-Shoulder Press, 178–79, **178–79**
  Side Lunge/Shoulder-to-Shoulder Press, 179, **179**
  Single-Arm, 84, **84**
  Staggered Stance Shoulder-to-Shoulder Press, 179, **179**
  Standing, 84, **84**
  Two-Hand, 119, **119**
Shoulder-to-Shoulder Press, 178–79, **178–79**
Shoveling, 152, **152**
Shrug, 69, **69**
Shucking, 153, **153**
Side Crunch Hip Thrust, 165, **165**
Side Lunge, 65, **65**, 174–75, **174–75**
Side Lunge Clean, 175, **175**
Side Lunge Shouldering, 143, **143**
Side Lunge/Shoulder-to-Shoulder Press, 179, **179**
Side Plank, 72, **72**
Side-to-Side Pickup, 171, **171**
Single-Arm Lateral Raise, 61, **61**
Single-Arm Push Press, 120, **120**
Single-Arm Shoulder Press, 84, **84**
Single-Arm Swing, 106–7, **106–7**, 107, 176, **176**
Single-Arm Triceps Kickback, 81, **81**
Single-Leg Calf Raise, 63, **63**
Single-Leg Good Morning, 169, **169**
Single-Leg Romanian Deadlift, 58, **58**, 100, **100**
Single-Leg Row, 76, **76**, 99, **99**, 180–81, **180–81**
Single-Leg Straight-Leg Deadlift, 59, **59**
Single-Leg Woodchop, 79, **79**
Six-Point Zenith, 105, **105**
SMR, 227

Snatch
    dumbbell, 86–87, **86–87**
    kettlebell, 110–11, **110–11**
    Rotating, 144, **144**
    sandbag, 144, **144**
    Two-Hand, 111, **111**
Soleus, 29
Sots, 121, **121**
Spinal erectors, 32
Squat, 54–55, **54–55**
    Bear Hug, 139, **139**
    Bulgarian Isometric, 55, **55**
    Front, 53, **53**
    Goblet, 126–27, **126–27**
    Good Morning, 169, **169**
    Jump, 55, **55**
    Pistol, 128–29, **128–29**
    Wide-Stance Bear Hug, 139,
        139
    Wide-Stance Goblet, 127, **127**
    Zercher, 145, **145**
    Zercher Squat and Press, 145,
        145
Staggered Stance Bent-Over
    Row, 181, **181**
Staggered Stance Clean and
    Press, 158, **158**
Staggered Stance Shoulder-to-
    Shoulder Press, 179, **179**
Standard Crunch, 147, **147**
Standing Shoulder Press, 84, **84**
Standing Twist, 73, **73**
Stepup, 74–75, **74–75**
    Crossover, 75, **75**
Straight-Leg Deadlift, 59, **59**
Strawberry, 40
Strength
    building with dumbbells, 12
    functional, 5, 16
    workouts for strength and
        mass
        Dumbbell Muscle Builder,
            229–37
        Kettlebell Muscle Builder,
            238–46
        Sandbag Muscle Builder,
            247–55
Suitcase Carry, 103, **103**

Sumo Deadlift, 57, **57**
Swing
    exercises
        dumbbell exercises, 197
        kettlebell exercises, 198
        sandbag exercises, 199
    muscles that help, 32–33
        abdominals, 32
        hip flexors, 33
        lower back, 32
Swing (exercise)
    Alternating Single-Arm, 107,
        107
    Double, 109, **109**
    Double-Arm, 108–9, **108–9**
    Half-Turn, 109, **109**
    kettlebell, 14
    sandbag, 176, **176**
    Single-Arm, 106–7, **106–7**, 107,
        176, **176**
    Walking, 109, **109**

T

Tabata, 204, 206, 222–26
Tactical Lunge, 124, **124–25**
Tate Press, 79, **79**
Testosterone
    boost with Kettlebell Swings,
        111
    decrease with dehydration, 40
Thirst, 40–41
Thruster, 127, **127**
Tools. *See also* Dumbbell(s);
        Kettlebell(s); Sandbag
    benefits of, 9–17
    choosing, 19–25
    making your own gear, 24
T-Pushup, 67, **67**
T-Raise, Lateral, 61, **61**
Transverse abdominis, 32
Transverse plane, 5–6
Trapezius, 29
Triceps brachii, 28
Triceps Extension
    Lying, 80, **80**
    Overhead, 82, **82**

Triceps Kickback
    Single-Arm, 81, **81**
    Two-Arm, 81, **81**
Triglycerides, lowering with
        blueberries, 95
Turkish Getup
    kettlebell, 132–33, **132–33**
    sandbag, 166–67, **166–67**
Two-Arm Push Press, 120, **120**
Two-Arm Row, 76, **76**
Two-Arm Triceps Kickback, 81,
        81
Two-Hand Shoulder Press, 119,
        119
Two-Hand Snatch, 111, **111**

U

Ultimate Sandbag Training
        System, 25
Unbalanced training, 4
Unilateral training, 10–11
Universal, 21
Upper body pull exercises
    dumbbell exercises, 197
    kettlebell exercises, 198
    sandbag exercises, 199
Upper body push exercises
    dumbbell exercises, 197
    kettlebell exercises, 198
    sandbag exercises, 199
Urine, color of, 40

V

Vastus intermedius, 28
Vastus lateralis, 28
Vastus medialis, 28
Vertical loading, 229
Vertical Single-Leg Row, 181, **181**

W

Walking Lunge, 65, **65**
Walking Swing, 109, **109**

Wall Drill, 104, **104**

Warmup, 194

Water, 40–41

Weight loss from water loss, 41

Whey protein shake, 39–40

    Bananas and Almonds, 39

    The Juicer, 40

    Strawberry and Banana, 40

Wide-Stance Bear Hug Squat, 139, **139**

Wide-Stance Goblet Squat, 127, **127**

Windmill, 134–35, **134–35**

    Double, 135, **135**

Woodchop, 78–79, **78–79**

Workouts

    building your own, 193–201

        Beginner 3-Day Workout, 195

        exercise type cheat sheet, 197–99

        Intermediate 4-Day Workout, 196

        Intermediate 3-Day Workout, 195

        muscle building basics for, 201

        order of exercises, 201

        points to keep in mind, 200

drinking as you exercise, 40–41

jumping rope between exercises, 162

kickstarters for movement mastery

    The Kettlebell Shredder, 204–7

    The Sandstorm, 208–12

length of, 201

metabolic training plans

    Dumbbell Fat Blaster, 213–21

    Kettlebell Fat Blaster, 222–26

    Sandbag Fat Blaster, 227–28

number per week, 201

1-rep rule, 194

1-Week Test Drives, 187–90

    dumbbell, 188–89

    kettlebell, 189

    sandbag, 190

for performance

    Dumbbell Performance Booster, 256–68

    Kettlebell Performance Booster, 269–71

    Sandbag Performance Booster, 272–81

pre- and postworkout eating plan, 37

for strength and mass

    Dumbbell Muscle Builder, 229–37

    Kettlebell Muscle Builder, 238–46

    Sandbag Muscle Builder, 247–55

varying, 201

warming up, 194

Wrist extensors and wrist flexors, 30

Y

Yates Row, 99, **99**

Z

Zercher Squat, 145, **145**

Zercher Squat and Press, 145, **145**

Zottman Curl, 47, **47**